BOOST YOUR
IMMUNE
SYSTEM

Other books by Patrick Holford

The Optimum Nutrition Bible
100% Health
Say No to Heart Disease
Balancing Hormones Naturally (with Kate Neil)
The Whole Health Manual
Elemental Health
How to Protect Yourself from Pollution
The Better Pregnancy Diet
Say No to Arthritis
The Fatburner Diet
Living Food
Mental Health and Illness – The Nutrition Connection

Other books by Jennifer Meek

Immune Power
Side Earth Syndrome

BOOST YOUR
IMMUNE
SYSTEM

JENNIFER MEEK & PATRICK HOLFORD

PIATKUS

© 1998 by Jennifer Meek and Patrick Holford

First published in 1998 by
Judy Piatkus (Publishers) Ltd
5 Windmill Street, London W1T 2JA
www.piatkus.co.uk

Reprinted 1999, 2000 (three times), 2003 (twice), 2004

The moral rights of the authors has been asserted

A catalogue record for this book is available from the British Library

ISBN 0 7499 1864 0

Designed by Paul Saunders

Typeset by Phoenix Photosetting, Chatham, Kent
Printed and bound in Great Britain by
Mackays of Chatham PLC, Chatham, Kent

CONTENTS

ACKNOWLEDGEMENTS

This book would not have been possible without the support of our families who put up with our absences, early mornings and late nights. Our thanks go to Pam Self for her help with research, Erica White for contributing the chapter on Candida, Peter Sofroniou for contributing the chapter on AIDS, and to the many scientists who have helped us access the latest research. Finally, our thanks to Natalie Savona for her editing and to Heather Rocklin and her team at Piatkus for their editorial advice, support, encouragement and assistance.

GUIDE TO ABBREVIATIONS AND MEASURES

1 gram (g) = 1000 milligrams (mg) = 1,000,000 micrograms (mcg or μg). Most vitamins are measured in milligrams or micrograms. Vitamins A, D and E are also measured in International Units (iu), a measurement designed to standardise the different forms of these vitamins which have different potencies.

1 mcg of retinol (mcg RE) = 3.3iu of vitamin A (RE = Retinol Equivalents)

1mcg RE of beta-carotene = 6mcg of beta-carotene

100iu of vitamin D = 2.5mcg

100iu of vitamin E = 67mg

1 pound (lb) = 16 ounces (oz)   2.2 lb = 1 kilogram (kg)

In this book calories means kilocalories (kcal)

REFERENCES AND FURTHER SOURCES OF INFORMATION

Hundreds of references from respected scientific literature have been used in writing this book. Details of specific studies referred to are listed on pages 169–72, together with further reading suggestions. Other supporting research for statements made is available from the Lamberts Library at the Institute for Optimum Nutrition (ION) (see page 173). Members are free to visit and study there. ION also offers information services, including literature search and library search facilities, for those readers who want to access scientific literature on specific subjects. On page 166 you will also find a Recommended Reading list which suggests the best books to read if you wish to dig deeper into the topics covered in each chapter.

HOW TO USE THIS BOOK

Here is an outline of this book to help you on your journey through the wonderful world of the immune system.

Part 1 shows to what extent your diet, lifestyle and environment may be affecting your immune system, and enables you to assess your own immune power.

Part 2 helps you to understand what the immune system is all about. It's a complex defence mechanism, but don't be put off by all the unfamilar words used to describe the different kinds of immune cells and their functions. The detail is there for those who want to go into depth; otherwise a light read will give you a good understanding of how your immune system works.

Part 3 explains the six main factors in keeping your immune system strong and healthy.

Part 4 gives you the latest information on how to deal with immune-related problems.

Part 5 gives you practical information about how to achieve optimum nutrition as a means to boosting your immunity and overall health.

Have a good journey and we wish you well in putting this information into practice in your life.

PART 1

ARE YOU IMMUNE?

CHAPTER 1

....

IMMUNITY IN CRISIS

When you are younger it is easy to fool yourself into believing that all those degenerative and life-threatening diseases will only happen to other people. But are you really immune to both minor and major infections and will cancer pass you by? Are you free from allergies and do you rarely suffer from a cold? If you want to answer yes, then you're reading the right book. Our purpose is to give you the knowledge to boost your immune system, to keep you free from disease, to feel better, perform better, look better and last longer.

This is timely advice because mankind may be on the brink of a worldwide crisis of immunity if the current trends in immune-related disease continue. Consider these facts:

- **By the year 2017 your chance of getting cancer is predicted to be greater than 50 per cent.**[1] Take breast cancer, for example. Currently, one in 12 women in the USA and one in eight in the UK develop breast cancer, and the numbers are rising. It is occurring more frequently and earlier in women's lives than it was a decade ago. The prediction is that by 2017 a woman's risk of developing cancer will be over 50 per cent and a man's over 65 per cent, with one in four men expected to get prostate cancer. We are currently losing, not winning, the cancer war.

- **Deaths from infectious diseases have doubled in a decade.**[2] In both the US and the UK the number of infections is dramatically on the increase. A survey of all deaths in the US between 1980 and 1992 revealed an alarming 58 per cent increase in deaths from infectious diseases.

- **Deaths from infectious diseases between the ages of 25 and 44 are up six-fold.** This is only partly due to the increased number of deaths from HIV infection. Deaths from respiratory infections alone increased by 20 per cent. According to Spence Galbraith, former Director of the Communicable Diseases Surveillance Centre, 'The rate of change of human infection appears to be increasing. It is now recognised that it can only be a matter of time until the next microbial menace to our species emerges amongst us.'[3]

- **A million people die each year from food poisoning.**[4] The growing incidence of disease caused by bugs in food, now second only to the common cold in some Western countries, may be one knock-on effect of the global use of around 50,000 tons of antibiotics each year.

- **50,000 tons of antibiotics are used each year throughout the world on humans, animals or plants.** In the UK alone, doctors write over 50 million prescriptions for antibiotics annually – roughly one per person per year.[5] Not only are antibiotics intestinal irritants, wiping out healthy intestinal bacteria that can take over six months to be restored, but their widespread use is leading to the development of drug-resistant strains of life-threatening bacteria, from staphylococci to mycobacterium tuberculosis and streptococci (responsible for most sore throats). The risk of a recurrent ear infection is five times higher in children treated with antibiotics.

- **One in three people suffer from allergies,** showing increased weaknesses in our immune systems.

- **We suffer, on average, three colds or bouts of flu a year,** the severity depending on the strength of the person's immune system. Each year, around 3000 people die from flu; during flu epidemics, the number can increase to 30,000.

The concept that germs cause disease (proved by Louis Pasteur in the nineteenth century) generated the idea that disease could be beaten and health restored by destroying the outside agent. And so we entered the era of a 'drug for a bug' – based on the belief that disease is a spanner in the works, caused by something that needs destroying, usually by using drugs. While this approach has produced some very positive results, the concept of 'combat medicine' is failing to provide much-needed new breakthroughs for most of the health problems we face today. The alternative is to boost your immune system.

Think of your immune system as your own personal medical team, skilled in the art of healing, always on call, and always there to take preventative measures to avert a crisis. Whether you are trying to prevent or cure an illness, your immune system is your main line of defence. It is worth looking after it so that it can serve you reliably and allow you to enjoy a happy, healthy life. Modern living, however, tends to do just the opposite – stressing, rather than strengthening, the immune army.

Within a relatively short period of time, we have dramatically changed our food, air, water and movement, in fact our whole way of living. We expect our bodies to adapt quickly, to find new ways of disposing of, or storing safely, all the 7000 new chemicals they are exposed to – pesticides, food additives, drugs, domestic detergents and other chemicals. Yet these have to be detoxified within us if they are to do no harm.

Nutrients found naturally in our food are often no longer

sufficient to enable our immune systems to cope efficiently with the increasing onslaught. Many people, overweight or not, take in more calories than they need. At the same time, we require more nutrients to help us cope with the extra pollution and stress. In food manufacture and preparation, however, nutrients are processed out of food, leaving us with nutrient-deficient products loaded with empty calories.

As you can already gather, there are many enemies to a healthy, efficient immune system and you cannot avoid them all. As in any war, the fewer enemies you have attacking you at any one time, the more likely you are to remain on top. How many can you identify and eliminate or reduce? Are there any others that you need to add to your own list, perhaps as a result of your occupation or where you live? The best you can do is try to minimise these enemies and boost your immune system to cope with the rest.

Listed below are some of the main enemies of the immune system:

- Smoke (tobacco and other – e.g. chimneys, incinerators, etc)

- Stress

- Pollution (busy roads, aeroplane flight paths, industry, etc)

- Pesticides

- Radiation

- Carcinogenic chemicals (industrial or domestic)

- Drugs (legal, illegal, medical); these all require medical supervision for reduction or elimination – do not try it alone

- Food additives (especially colours and flavours)

- Incorrect balance of food (e.g. too much salt, fat or sugar)

- Accidents

- Obesity or starvation

- Poor mineral balance

- Poor vitamin balance

- Inappropriate exercise

- Genetic defects

- Infections (from bacteria, viruses, fungi, protozoa, worms, etc)

- Negative attitude to life

- Unhappiness

WHY YOUR IMMUNE SYSTEM NEEDS BOOSTING

Here are some good reasons for boosting your immune system:

1. Your immune system determines how fast you age.

2. Your immune system fights off the viruses, bacteria and other organisms which try to attack you and cause illness, from the common ones that cause colds and thrush, to the rarer but often deadly ones like meningitis, Legionnaire's disease and AIDS.

3. Your immune system has the power to destroy cancer cells as they are formed.

4. Your immune system empties your body's dustbin every day, getting rid of dead cells, dead invaders and toxic chemicals.

5. Your immune system offers protection from radiation and chemical pollutants.

6. Left to deteriorate, your immune system could lose control and cause allergy problems or auto–immune diseases like arthritis.

7. With a struggling immune system, you are ill more often, more seriously, and for longer.

8. With a strong immune system, you are almost invincible and should be able to lead a long, healthy and active life.

Essentially, life is for living and giving, for learning and loving, for achieving and enjoying, and no one wants to waste more time than they have to being sick.

CHAPTER 2

....

HOW STRONG IS YOUR
IMMUNE SYSTEM?

It's your body – it's been with you since before you were
born – but how well do you know it? How well do you listen to it? Just as we all have different fingerprints, so we all
have different physical, nutritional and emotional requirements, and different early warning signs that something is
amiss. Your body will tell you if it is getting too many toxic
minerals or not enough nutritional ones, if it is under stress, or
not getting enough exercise or sleep, or if it is being invaded
by viruses or bacteria. But do you listen to it and understand
what it is saying?

It is important to get to know what the healthy you is like
and to be aware of any slight changes. How loud does your
immune system have to shout before you take any notice?
The earlier you recognise the symptoms, the faster you can
take corrective action and the more likely you are to avoid
becoming really ill. Use the list of early warning signs overleaf
as a checklist. If your score is high, it's time to give your
immune system a boost.

Single symptoms show localised problems or changes
which may or may not be significant. For instance, a painful
ear could mean an ear infection which, if not treated, could
become serious, whereas feeling ravenously hungry after a
long walk in the country is a perfectly normal request by the
body for more fuel rather than a warning of a tapeworm

inhabiting your gut! Combinations of symptoms are often more significant. Either way, pay attention to your body's messages and try to supply its needs.

Early Warning Signs of an Immune System in Trouble

Do you notice any changes in the following?

Hair   Fall, texture, dry or greasy, colour, lack of growth?

Head   Dull ache, pain on movement, flushing or burning sensations, feelings of floating, fogginess, dizziness?

Eyes   Yellowed whites, bloodshot, itchy, stinging, dull not sparkling, pain on movement from side to side, watery, change in vision, tiredness?

Ears   Itchy, painful, noises inside, sounds appearing far away whilst own voice is loud, flaking skin?

Nose   Running, itching, sore, congested, difficulty breathing, loss of smell, sneezing?

Mouth   Bad taste, bad breath, coated tongue, ulcers, loss of taste, bleeding gums, bad teeth, sore tongue, difficulty chewing, change in quantity of saliva?

Neck   Stiffness or pain on movement?

Throat   Sore, painful to swallow, swollen glands?

Digestive tract   Indigestion, gas, burning sensations, bloatedness, pain, constipation, diarrhoea?

Muscles   Weakened, painful, numb, tingling, flabby, tense, easily injured?

Joints Stiffness, weakness, tremors, swelling, pain?

Skin Spots, rashes, colour change, dry flaky, blotchy, new or altered moles or body hair, dull, tight, flabby, bloated, body odour?

Nails Ridged, brittle, white spots, blue-tinged, split?

Energy levels Higher, lower, intermittent, erratic, hyper-active, dependent on food, coffee or other stimulant intake?

Sleep Poor, broken, heavy, restless, excessive sweating, altered dreaming?

Mental state Poor concentration, poor memory, lack of interest, forgetfulness?

Hunger Ravenously hungry, off food, food cravings?

Mood Depressed, sad, up and down, irritable, frustrated, despairing?

HOW DOES YOUR IMMUNE SYSTEM IMPROVE YOUR HEALTH?

Health is defined by the World Health Organisation as a state of complete physical, mental, emotional and social well-being, not merely the absence of disease or infirmity. By this ideal standard most of us are in various states of 'unhealthiness' for much of our lives. However, although we will never reach perfection, we are all capable of striving for excellence and thereby avoiding a lot of illness.

There are always plenty of disease-causing bacteria, viruses, fungi and other organisms lurking, either in our bodies or in the environment, waiting for an opportunity to attack a susceptible human. They are a part of life we cannot avoid but we do have a system for coping with them – armies of immune cells which recognise these invaders, attack them and we hope, destroy them before they destroy us. If our personal immune system is overworked, inefficient or undernourished, it cannot sustain an army able to recognise the enemy and destroy it – that's when we develop disease. How long the disease affects us depends on how long it takes for the immune system to become effective and fight back.

By maintaining our immune system in peak condition, it is possible, at best, to avoid symptoms of illness completely and, at worst, to put together an effective fighting force quickly so that the illness is less severe. The immune system can also destroy cancer cells. We all generate these abnormal cells but usually keep them under control. It is when they are formed too quickly for the immune system to keep up with that cancer becomes a problem.

Similarly, as long as the immune system is working correctly, there is no problem with auto-immune diseases. It is only when the immune system goes wrong and does not recognise itself any more that auto-immune diseases occur, when the 'army' starts attacking the body's own cells as well as those of its enemies.

Check the Strength of Your Immune System

The following signs, symptoms and lifestyle factors will indicate how strong your immune system is likely to be.

The more times you answer yes, the more strain your immune system is likely to be under. Score 1 for each 'yes' answer.

Health

- Do you get more than three colds a year? **YES / NO**
- Do you find it hard to shift an infection (cold or otherwise)? **YES / NO**
- Are you prone to thrush or cystitis? **YES / NO**
- Do you generally take antibiotics twice or more each year? **YES / NO**
- Have you had a major personal loss in the past year? **YES / NO**
- Is there any history of cancer in your family? **YES / NO**
- Do you take any drugs or medicines? **YES / NO**
- Do you have an inflammatory disease such as eczema, asthma or arthritis? **YES / NO**
- Do you suffer from hay fever? **YES / NO**
- Do you suffer from allergy problems? **YES / NO**

Diet

- Do you drink more than 1 unit of alcohol a day? **YES / NO**
- Do you drink less than 1 litre of water a day (including that in drinks)? **YES / NO**
- Do you eat more than 1 tablespoon of sugar a day? **YES / NO**
- Do you rarely eat raw fruit and vegetables? **YES / NO**
- Do you rarely take supplements? **YES / NO**
- Do you eat a lot of refined, processed or convenience foods? **YES / NO**
- Do you need something to get you going in the morning or at regular intervals during the day, like tea or coffee or cigarettes? **YES / NO**
- Do you often feel drowsy or sleepy during the day, or after meals? **YES / NO**
- Do you eat meat more than five times a week? **YES / NO**
- Do you eat a lot of processed, snack foods in between or instead of meals? **YES / NO**

Lifestyle

- Do you spend less than one hour exposed to natural light each day? **YES / NO**
- Do you take very little exercise? **YES / NO**
- Is your job sedentary? **YES / NO**
- Do you smoke? **YES / NO**
- Do you live or work in a smoky environment? **YES / NO**
- Do you sleep badly or wake up with your mind racing? **YES / NO**
- Are you unhapy with any major aspect of your life? **YES / NO**
- Do you easily get upset, angry, anxious or irritable? **YES / NO**
- Are you overweight? **YES / NO**
- Do you often eat on the run or under stress? **YES / NO**

If you score …

20 or more You need to make some considerable changes to your diet and lifestyle if you want to achieve a strong immune system that will keep you consistently healthy. This book will give you clear guidance. You may also wish to consider seeing a nutrition consultant who can speed up your transition to maximum immune power (see Useful Addresses).

10 or more You are average but who wants to be average? Look at your 'yes' answers and find ways of changing your diet and lifestyle to turn these into 'no' answers. This book will tell you how.

Less than 10 You are doing well and are likely to have a reasonably strong immune system. To fine-tune your health, take note of your 'yes' answers and find ways of changing your diet and lifestyle to turn these into 'no' answers.

PART 2

UNDERSTANDING YOUR IMMUNE SYSTEM

CHAPTER 3

HOW THE IMMUNE SYSTEM WORKS

Immunity literally means 'being exempt from getting something'. Your immune system is very complex and has to be finely tuned to be able to destroy anything which threatens your body.

THE ROLE OF YOUR IMMUNE SYSTEM

Keeping a Balance

When you are in good health, everything is in balance – everything is working in harmony with everything else, resulting in a healthy whole. When you are sick, the balance is lost and your immune system battles conscientiously to restore it. If it succeeds, you get well again. If it does not, other influences may take advantage of the upset system and join the battle, causing further imbalance. As long as your immune system stays in control, the battle will eventually be won and order will be restored.

Fighting Infections

Bacteria, viruses, fungi, parasites and worms freely inhabit our world. There is no way of avoiding them completely in normal life so the key is to have a balanced inner environment.

Coming into contact with a disease-causing bacterium does not automatically mean that it will take over. We constantly live with the fungus that causes thrush, for example, or the bugs that cause pneumonia. But most of us have a balanced immune system that keeps them under control. However, taking a lot of antibiotics that kill our friendly bacteria allows the irritant fungus (not affected by the antibiotics) to grow into spaces where the friendly bugs would normally be, resulting in thrush. Likewise, if our immune system has been fighting a serious disease and the body's defences are low, the pneumonia bugs can seize their opportunity and attack, causing pneumonia.

Many diseases, including the common cold, are infections – we should try not to spread them, in particular to the very young, the sick and the elderly. It is a poor friend who has an infection yet goes to hospital to visit someone who has just had a baby or has undergone surgery. Keep your unfriendly bugs to yourself!

Making Exceptions

Our bodies cannot destroy everything foreign that enters them: food, for example, is essential for life even though it is 'foreign' or non-self. The gut's immune system is therefore adapted so that we can take such material into it. For instance, we can usually eat an egg with no ill effects, but if it were injected straight into our bloodstream the immune system there would attack it immediately.

In order for us to reproduce, 'foreign' sperm has to enter the female body. The sperm (which is non-self) therefore has to have in-built local immune suppressors to prevent the female's immune system rejecting it. And, of course, a pregnant woman's whole immune system has to adapt dramatically in order to allow a completely different body to live inside her for nine months.

Many bacteria are unfriendly, but not all; some are necessary for our normal everyday existence and carry out important functions, so it is very important that our immune system does not attack these. When our friendly gut bugs are destroyed by antibiotics, we are left open to attack by fungi and other pathogens (harmful organisms). We need our friendly neighbourhood bugs in the gut, on the skin, and in our mucous membranes to stop the foreigners settling in and changing the environment to their own advantage – and our disadvantage.

Keeping the Peace

At a more fundamental level, 'civil war' within the body must be avoided – the immune system must not attack its own men (a difficult task when there are several million million of them, of many different sorts). It is also important that weapons intended for use against invaders do not accidentally destroy our own defenders; such weapons need to be carefully stored and disarmed during 'peacetime'.

TYPES OF IMMUNITY

Our bodies provide two main types of immunity. Antibodies, for example, target particular invaders, providing specific immunity. Other factors, like our own physical barriers (such as skin and mucous membranes) act more generally, giving indiscriminate, non-specific immunity.

Non-Specific Immunity

Physical Barriers

Our first line of defence is in the form of physical barriers that protect us from attack, the most obvious being the skin.

Secretions from its glands (such as salt in sweat) contain anti-fungal and anti-bacterial substances that protect the outer layer. We also have many friendly bacteria on the skin's surface that prevent invasion by less friendly ones. As long as our skin is intact, we are relatively safe; if, however, the skin has a wound, there is a risk of infection.

Obviously, in order to breathe, eat, excrete and reproduce, we have to have entrances into our bodies. These, in turn, have special skin surfaces and secretions that protect them. The damp, mucous membranes of the nose and respiratory tract, for example, along with the hairs and cilia (microscopic hairs), trap many would-be invaders.

Some well-known respiratory bugs, like the ones that cause flu, interfere with the sweeping action of the cilia, which is why they are so successful at making us ill. There are no cilia in the gut, but mucus and peristalsis (the constant pushing movement of the gut) prevent much bacterial growth; the churning action and acidity of the stomach also inhibit infection. Infection occurs when the mucous membrane is damaged or when peristalsis slows down, and can also be caused by food poisoning.

Skin and mucous membranes, as well as the blood brain barrier and (before we are born) the placenta, all prevent free exchange of material and so, to a degree, protect us from harmful agents. Coughing, sneezing and crying also get rid of potentially harmful substances.

Temperature

Many of the bugs that make us ill are very fussy about temperature: for example, the bacillus that causes TB in humans will not infect cold-blooded animals. Likewise, the bugs which cause gonorrhoea are killed above 40°C; so, before antibiotics became available, raising the body temperature was a common treatment for this condition.

Many of the body's own immune cells work better at a temperature above normal which is why fever often accompanies infection. Trying to lower a temperature can therefore put our immune cells at a disadvantage, as mild fever aids the immune response. A mild fever should therefore be left to run its course, so it can do its job, just as the old phrase 'sweating out' a sickness implies. However, a very high temperature, when the body appears to have lost control, must be lowered or it could be dangerous in itself.

Biochemical Barriers

We also make chemicals inside us which destroy unwanted bugs and other substances. (Their effect is general, not specific to any one kind of bug.) Blood, eye fluids and many of our cells carry an enzyme called lysozyme which is one such chemical and can destroy bacteria.

Interferon is an anti-viral agent, secreted by most tissue cells throughout the body (as long as they have significant vitamin C and manganese), which acts against any virus that it finds lurking about. It prevents a virus from multiplying inside our cells, probably by closing down its power source; it can also prevent neighbouring cells from being infected.

The ability to make interferon is coded in our genes, our inherited material. Indeed the human interferon gene can now be synthesised. This could obviously be very useful in medicine, although it is not the whole answer to the elimination of harmful viruses.

We also have a group of proteins in our blood which come together, when stimulated, to bring about the destruction of unwanted material. This is known as the complement system and it seems to trigger inflammation. In order to prevent their uncontrolled attack, the complement proteins are usually found separated in the blood. It is only when they come together in the correct order, stimulated by a threatening situation, that they cause destruction. It is rather like taking a gun apart to prevent it going off by accident and only putting it together when there is something to shoot.

Blood, sweat, tears and other body fluids (such as bile salts and essential fatty acids in the intestines) contain other biochemically active anti-bug substances.

Species

Not all living things are susceptible to all disease-causing organisms. For example, you never see a dog with measles because the germs that cause this illness do not affect dogs. The rabies virus, however, will attack both man and dog once it gets under skin.

Likewise, rats are not susceptible to the diphtheria bacteria and can live quite happily in a sewer, whilst guinea pigs are highly susceptible and would not survive long in such an environment. The myxomatosis virus favours rabbits, whilst the bacteria for leprosy and syphilis prefer man. By virtue of being human, we can safely say that we will not suffer from fowl pox or potato blight – we are naturally immune.

Genetics

There are some illnesses which are genetically determined. Most of us, for example, do not suffer from haemophilia. It is not an infection; you cannot catch it; you cannot make it go away by altering diet or exercise. If it is not in your genes you will not get it.

Specific Immunity

Parts of the immune system act against particular bugs or conditions. Specific immunity, as it is known, is usually divided into active and passive immunity and both are further divided into natural and artificial immunity.

Passive Immunity

This is when antibodies or anti-toxins are transferred from an immune person to a non-immune person. This happens naturally when immunity is passed from mother to child via the placenta or in colostrum (in breast milk). Artificially, passive immunity may be used to treat tetanus, snake bite or those with immune-deficient diseases. Neither natural nor artificial passive immunity lasts long: once the substance passed on to the non-immune person is used up, the beneficial effects are lost.

Active Immunity

This is when the body's own immune cells recognise a specific bug or substance and react to it. They can then remember and deal with the problem on subsequent occasions. Natural active immunity occurs during infection, and we gain artificial active immunity when we are immunised (see Chapter 17 for more on vaccinations).

NUTRITIONAL SUPPORT

As you will already have gathered, the functioning of the immune system is very dependent on specific nutrients. Our production of natural antibiotics and complement proteins, and the ability of our cells to carry out, engulf and digest invaders are all dependent on vitamin C, so increased consumption of this vitamin at the time of infection (rather than later when symptoms start to show) is crucial. Taking vitamin C at the time of infection immediately increases your level of protection; taken a day or so later, it will be far less effective.

Our production of complement proteins is dependent on calcium and magnesium, whilst our interferon production depends on the mineral manganese. Calcium is also needed to produce a fever, which, as we have seen, in its mild form aids our immune soldiers. All three nutrients are commonly deficient in our modern-day, refined diet.

So our immune system can be impaired by something as simple as vitamin C deficiency. The benefits of good nutrition for the immune system are explained in depth in Chapters 8 and 9.

....

CHAPTER 4

THE IMMUNE ARMY AND THE BATTLEGROUND

Immunological battles can occur anywhere in the body – against invading organisms, 'foreign' proteins and even our own misbehaving cells, such as cancer cells. To fight off any enemies, we have a fixed defence framework, called the lymphatic system (shown in Figure 1) which works alongside other parts of the body such as the bone marrow, thymus and spleen. The complex workings of the immune system are largely controlled by the pituitary and adrenal glands.

THE LYMPHATIC SYSTEM

This is a network of vessels which branches throughout the entire body and contains a clear fluid called lymph. Unlike the blood system, there is no pump to force the lymph around. This fluid is instead moved by muscle contraction; hence the importance of exercise in preventing a sluggish immune system.

The lymph nodes, or glands, lie on the lymphatic vessels and are areas of high immunological activity – active battle-grounds when war is underway. As you can see from Figure 1, the body is, for defence purposes, divided into six areas. Each area has its own nodes (where much of the fighting takes place); these nodes become the 'enlarged glands' which appear in many infections. Each area tries to keep such

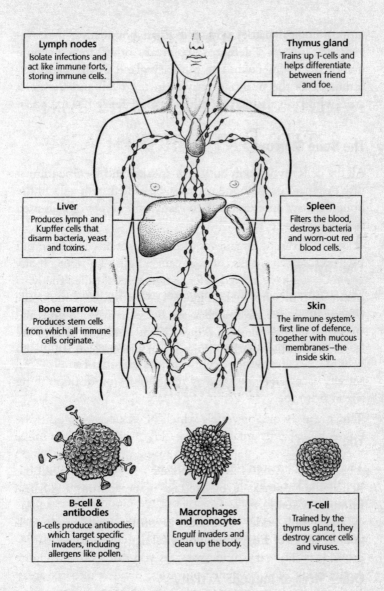

Lymph nodes
Isolate infections and act like immune forts, storing immune cells.

Thymus gland
Trains up T-cells and helps differentiate between friend and foe.

Liver
Produces lymph and Kupffer cells that disarm bacteria, yeast and toxins.

Spleen
Filters the blood, destroys bacteria and worn-out red blood cells.

Bone marrow
Produces stem cells from which all immune cells originate.

Skin
The immune system's first line of defence, together with mucous membranes—the inside skin.

B-cell & antibodies
B-cells produce antibodies, which target specific invaders, including allergens like pollen.

Macrophages and monocytes
Engulf invaders and clean up the body.

T-cell
Trained by the thymus gland, they destroy cancer cells and viruses.

Figure 1 – The Immune System

immunological battles within its own boundaries; if, however, the person's defences are weak, other areas become involved and infected. The pituitary gland in the brain co-ordinates all the immune activity in the head and the neck area, while the central core is the main defence headquarters.

The Bone Marrow

All the cells involved in both non-specific and specific immunity originate in the bone marrow. So-called stem cells in the bone marrow differentiate into many other types of cells used in the immune system.

The Thymus

The master gland of the immune system, the thymus, is situated behind the breast bone. It is very active before and around the time of birth, but begins to decrease in size and activity from puberty onwards. Growth hormone stimulates it, while sex hormones depress it. It is essential for all T cell activity (see page 30), and is responsible for distinguishing friend from foe.

The Spleen

The spleen, situated near the stomach, is made of lymph tissue that is specially designed to filter blood. It also destroys certain bacteria as well as worn-out red blood cells and plays an important part in specific immunity involving B cells (which produce antibodies, see page 31).

Other Sites of Immune Activity

Other areas of special importance in the immune system are scattered throughout the body. In the liver the Kupffer cells play a role in immunity, while elsewhere the tonsils, adenoids, appendix, Peyer's patches in the intestines, and others have a similar function.

THE BLOOD AND BLOOD CELLS

The blood is an important part of the defence system. It is made up of a clear yellow fluid (called plasma) and blood cells which are suspended in the fluid. Blood is pumped around the entire body by the heart. Major blood vessels branch into smaller ones and eventually into a network of fine capillaries so that the blood can reach every tissue. It takes oxygen all over the body from the lungs, and transports the waste carbon dioxide away. It carries food to every tissue and cleans up afterwards by taking waste to the kidneys and liver for eventual removal. It also distributes heat to all parts of the body.

Finally, the blood provides us with a mobile fighting force of white blood cells which are our main immune soldiers. When our systems are in good working order, we are able to synthesise around 2000 new immune cells every second. That's some fighting force, and would be quite a deterrent if germs had any brains! White blood cells or leukocytes are present in lymph as well as in the blood. Some can even squeeze into tissue when they are needed to fight an infection.

Platelets

Platelets are small fragments in the blood that are important for our defence because they can get stuck together and coagulate the blood when there is an injury, so preventing all 5 litres pouring out of the hole and leaving our bodies empty! The plasma contains a substance called fibrin which forms a mesh at the site of the wound, to which the platelets stick. There are between 150,000 and 400,000 platelets per cubic millimetre of blood.

Red Blood Cells

There are some 25 million million red blood cells or erythrocytes in the body of an adult man, or about 5 million per cubic millimetre. These are more like robots than soldiers because, two or three days before they mature and leave the bone marrow where they are formed, they squeeze out their nuclei; this removes their ability to divide again to form new cells, so they are destined for destruction about four months later.

After leaving the bone marrow they enter the bloodstream, where their role is really only to act as a vehicle for carrying oxygen around the body. They do, however, have suction pads or docking points on their surface. Should any of the 25 million million of them come across anything alien whilst they are on their oxygen delivery rounds, they can use these suction pads to arrest it and deliver it to one of the white blood cells.

White Blood Cells

There are three main types of white blood cell.

Granulocytes

Granulocytes are further divided into polymorphonuclear neutrophils (PMNs), eosinophils and basophils. The eosinophils and basophils make up at most 6 per cent of the total white blood cell count and are significant in allergies and worm infections. PMNs are very small cells and make up 50 to 70 per cent of the total white cell count. They are phagocytic, which means that they gobble up any foreign bacteria they come across.

Enzymes released from the PMNs bleach the alien to death, but are strong enough to digest the little PMNs as well. Pus found at the site of an infection is therefore a mixture of dead bacteria and the dead PMN army that has fought so hard to conquer the enemy.

Monocytes

Monocytes are much larger than red blood cells and PMNs, and are essentially the same as macrophages. Although less than 10 per cent of the total white blood cell count consists of macrophages, they are crucial. They eat anything that is rubbish or foreign, and clean our blood, tissues and lymph like efficient, selective vacuum cleaners. This means, in effect, that the whole of our body has guards posted around it whose sole purpose is to look for and get rid of any unwanted material.

Macrophages and other phagocytic cells in the blood and lymph feed on any of our cells which are dead or broken, and any rubbish or invaders. They get breakfast, lunch, dinner, snacks and midnight feasts, whilst protecting us from attacks.

Macrophages are also major chemical factories, capable of making at least 40 different enzymes and immune proteins needed for the destruction of enemies. Their peacetime chemical activities include making the enzymes necessary for blood clotting and fat transport.

They are not necessarily killed during an attack and they may live for some time. But, even in death, they are useful, as they are broken down, cannibal-style, by other macrophages and used as food.

Lymphocytes

Lymphocytes make up somewhere between 20 and 30 per cent of the total white cell count (depending on the degree of infection of the person at a given time). They are the most competent and versatile group of cells for getting rid of 'unwanted guests'. There are around one million million lymphocytes in the average adult body and the principal centres for their production are the lymph nodes, spleen, thymus, Peyer's patches, appendix and other lymphoid tissue.

Some lymphocytes have a memory system, so that, when a second or third invasion by the same kind of bug occurs, the immune system can move into action right away, instead of wasting time relearning old lessons. Because a re-infection can be tackled immediately, it is usually much milder than an initial attack. Lymphocytes have a special method of dividing rapidly when under attack; this means that they can produce reinforcements almost immediately and the person hardly knows that they have been under attack. This rapid division is very nutrient-dependent — for example, vitamin C levels are crucial. All lymphocytes can move around between tissues, lymph and the bloodstream, so body-wide distribution and memory are ensured. The two major types of lymphocytes are T cells and B cells.

T Lymphocytes

Not all T lymphocytes do the same jobs but all have passed through the thymus (the master immune computer) for programming before they are let loose on the body. Some are unarmed and cruise around on surveillance duty, whilst others carry deadly warheads. They provide the initial response to viruses, tumour cells and the rejection of transplants. But it takes three to four days after recognition of these for the T cells to get their act together and attack.

   T helper cells (TH or T4 cells) help other members of the immune army, but are not armed themselves. If there is an invader of questionable identity, these T helper cells decide whether it is a threat. They are also responsible for verifying an invasion and switching the immune system on. The human immunodeficiency virus that causes *AIDS* tends to invade these cells, leaving the victim with very few of these helper cells, and tricking the body into keeping the immune system switched off, even though there is a major invasion taking place.

   T suppressor cells (TS or T8 cells) switch off the immune system (both B and T cells) when an infection has passed and recovery is complete. Like the helper cells, the T suppressor cells are not armed.

   Cytotoxic T cells come complete with destructive

powers. Their special duty is to search out viruses, etc, which have hidden themselves inside our cells. Most of the body's immune army, when they come across a 'self' cell, recognise it and leave it alone, but the cytotoxic T cell has the ability to seek out and destroy any of the body cells that have a traitor within. They have very strong enzyme 'missiles' which break up and destroy the infected cell. Although they do have a specific target, there is bound to be some damage caused to surrounding cells by the use of such strong weapons.

Lymphokine–producing T cells also have missiles, but these are aimed at invaders which move in-between the body's own cells. Both these and the cytotoxic cells stimulate an increase in activity by the macrophages, as the lymphokines and other chemical weapons cause a lot of destruction which leaves a lot of dead cells and debris to be cleared away.

B Lymphocytes

B lymphocytes deal mainly with bacteria and viruses that have been encountered before. Attack by a B cell is thus very specific; furthermore, it often requires help from other immune cells. The task of a B cell is to take an invading bug into the tissues, where it ascertains its exact size and shape. It then tailor-makes a straitjacket, called an antibody, that will fit that bug and no other. Finally, it gets a production line going to manufacture thousands more of these antibodies which are released back into the body.

These, in turn, search out their targets like mini guided missiles and attach themselves to the bacteria. The invader becomes harmless and is held until the macrophages or PMNs come along to devour it.

ANTIBODIES

Each antibody is a Y-shaped protein with a clamp or straitjacket on each of the two top arms. Although they are made en masse in one of five basic patterns, the end product is tailored very specifically to one particular bug. The patterns for these antibodies are held in memory banks, so that they can be made to order immediately, should re-infection occur.

This is the principle upon which vaccination is based, whereby small quantities of a killed or altered bug are injected into the bloodstream so that antibodies can be made to match it. On subsequent infection by the same bug, the body can act right away and kill the bug before it has a chance to take hold and reproduce.

When first infected, it can take five days before the body produces an antibody response. Peak levels are then recorded after around 14 days. On re-infection, however, antibodies can often be detected within 48 hours, and they stay in the system much longer.

Antibodies are often referred to as immunoglobulins. The infecting agents, or antigens are presented to the B lymphocytes by the T lymphocytes, prompting the B cells to mature and produce one of five antibody patterns: IgG, IgA, IgM, IgD or IgE.

IgG

This is the most abundant antibody, making up 75 per cent of all those in blood plasma. It is most active in the blood, lymph and intestines. PMNs and macrophages have receptor sites for the IgG antibody and so can attach and eat the antibody and its captives when it is ready.

IgG is required by cells which are active in destroying cancer cells, although, unfortunately, the same cells are also involved in transplant rejection and auto-immune diseases. IgG is actively transported across the placenta and gives both the foetus and the newborn baby protection for up to six months. The infant usually starts making its own IgG at

around three months, which is when immunisation programmes often begin.

IgA

This type of antibody is found in blood serum and in the
mucous secretions of the respiratory, genito-urinary and intestinal tracts, where exposure to foreign substances is common.
Being proteins, immunoglobulins are liable to be digested by
the gut enzymes, but IgA can produce a secretion which gives
it some protection against this. In gastric juices, 80 per cent of
the immunoglobulins are IgA. IgA is often low in those who
suffer from respiratory and gastro-intestinal infections.

IgA's memory and specificity is poor in comparison with
the other antibodies, but this is necessary, particularly in the
gut, otherwise we could become irrevocably sensitised to
almost anything we ate – a boiled egg, for example. People
who suffer from food allergy problems probably have malfunctioning IgA; they become over-sensitive to certain foods
which, in any other person, would not be harmful. Hayfever
sufferers are similar; pollen is not really harmful in itself, but
some people have a violent reaction to these usually harmless
particles (see Chapter 7 on allergies).

IgM

IgM is the largest and most primitive immunoglobulin. Its
size makes it useful for picking up lots of small antigens,
which it can manage 10 at a time. It is particularly important
early on in any immune response.

IgD

Not a lot is known about IgD, but levels are high in kwash-
iorkor (a disease of malnutrition).

IgE

IgE is attracted to cells involved in allergic response and basophils (a type of granulocyte). It is associated with all forms of allergy, including hayfever, asthma, hives, itching, rhinitis, etc. People who suffer from allergies usually make too much IgE, and their allergic tendency can be passed on to their children, although the allergy may not take the same form or have the same symptoms.

A SUMMARY OF THE IMMUNE SYSTEM'S WEAPONS

Red blood cells merely arrest invaders and pass the 'prisoners' to the white blood cells to deal with.

There are several types of white blood cells:

- Macrophages and PMNs eat the enemy.

- Eosinophils and basophils cause inflammation and warn of infection.

- B lymphocytes only attack specific targets. They need one or two weeks to make a good supply of antibody and to remember their targets so that they can supply the antibody faster should there be a second attack.

- T lymphocytes regulate the immune system and decide whether it should go into battle or withdraw. Some T lymphocytes attack.

Finally, let's look at three terms that often cause confusion:

Antigens are anything which provokes an antibody response. Bugs which can cause disease are said to be antigenic because their presence in the body causes the B cells to make antibodies which coat and help to destroy invading bugs. An allergy provoking food is also an antigen.

Antibiotics are a sort of mercenary chemical force sometimes sent in by doctors to help combat a bacterial infection. Antibiotics are not made in the body, and should not be confused with antibodies – they are not the same thing at all.

CHAPTER 5

THE CAUSES AND CONSEQUENCES OF INFECTION

There is an underlying purpose for everything, including sickness. The usual purpose of physical or mental pain is to draw attention to an imbalance in the body which requires correction. Sickness is the body's way of warning us of an attack, usually from external forces, like germs. But sometimes it's telling us that we are doing something wrong which is causing us to malfunction.

When we are ill, our energy level drops because we are using energy to make more heat, which improves the activity of our immune cells as our temperature goes up. Our limbs ache or feel heavy because our available stores of calcium and magnesium go to aid defence, leaving our joints short of these essential minerals. We may also experience loss of appetite and digestive problems, because we don't have any energy to spare for digestion. We lose weight, because we use body stores for energy in the initial stages, rather than immediately digested food (which is often not digested properly at this time anyway). The tongue becomes coated and the skin condition deteriorates, because these are major sites for removal of toxins.

THE CAUSES OF INFECTION

There are several types of 'germ' in the air, on food, in water or anywhere waiting to attack susceptible humans: bacteria, viruses, parasites, protozoa and fungi. Successful bugs will live in or on us for a while, replicate or reproduce, and move on to new human hosts.

Bacterial Infection

Bacteria are the most well-known cause of infectious diseases. Some try to evade the immune system by forming a protective capsule around themselves, e.g. the streptococci which cause sore throats and the bacteria that cause flu, pneumonia and meningitis. (There are viruses that can cause these illnesses too.) Other bacteria have cell walls which are resistant to digestion by enzymes in our gut e.g. salmonella and the bacteria which cause TB (*Mycobacterium tuberculosis*) and leprosy (*Mycobacterium leprae*).

Other bacteria produce chemicals that attempt to immobilise the immune army. These include tetanus (*Clostridium tetani*), diphtheria (*Corynebacterium diphtheriae*) and cholera (*Vibrio cholerae*). The toxins they produce continue to do harm even after the bug has been killed. Some very successful bacteria, like Pseudomonas, Listeria and E. coli, only cause problems when the immune system is under par for some reason, e.g. immaturity, pregnancy, illness or old age. Antibiotic drugs are sometimes used to combat bacterial infection. However, not all bacteria have special properties and many can be dealt with very effectively by a competent immune system.

Viral Infection

Viruses are another common cause of infectious diseases. They are very small and therefore more difficult to study. As yet, there are no 'magic bullets' (like antibiotics) to destroy them, so it's all down to the immune system. Our first line of defence against the virus is interferon. This is in an inactive form in the body until it comes across a virus and its action is not specific. When it is activated by the presence of viral particles it makes a protein, which, in effect, stops the virus reproducing and so makes it ineffective. Interferon also stops the host (body) cell from reproducing, so that cell eventually dies too. It's very potent stuff, and highly dependent on sufficient vitamin C and the mineral manganese.

Whilst the viruses that cause diseases like mumps, measles, smallpox, herpes, polio, typhus and yellow fever are in our blood, our antibodies can attack them. The success of the virus depends on its ability to get inside a host cell, where it can use the host's DNA to replicate itself. In effect, they play one of the oldest tricks in the book – the Trojan horse. Once they get this far, the only immune cell capable of recognising and destroying them is the cytotoxic T cell.

Some viruses stay in the body even after obvious infection has passed, and they can be re-activated at a later date, causing the same or sometimes different symptoms. The herpes viruses, which cause cold sores, are a good example of this. And the chicken pox virus can present itself again as shingles at a later date, when the body's defences are low.

Rhinoviruses (which cause colds and flu) are so successful because they constantly change the recognition code on their surface. As fast as medical science finds a cure for one type of flu, the bug changes and researchers have to start all over again on the new form.

Other Infectious Agents

There are less than 20 protozoa that cause disease in man and they aren't much of a problem in this country. When they do strike they are difficult to combat because they have similar cells to us, so something that will attack them is liable to attack and destroy our own cells too. The most formidable ones are the insect-borne protozoa which cause malaria (*Plasmodium*), sand-fly fever (*Leishmania*) and sleeping sickness (*Trypanosomes*).

Toxocariasis – passed to humans via cats or dogs – is the main parasitic infection that gives cause for concern in the UK. (The worms need a host other than man to reproduce in.) Pets should be wormed regularly because the Toxicara larvae burrow into blood vessels in the intestine, then go to the liver and sometimes get into the lungs, eye or brain where they can cause irrevocable damage.

Athlete's foot, ringworm and thrush are probably the most common fungal infections. Candida (the fungus that causes thrush), in particular, is increasing rapidly. This is possibly partly due to the use of antibiotics which kill all the good bacteria in the body as well as the unwanted ones, leaving the fungi unaffected. Unless you are very quick to do something about it, the fungi are able to reproduce and take up all the space that was previously inhabited by good bacteria. After a course of antibiotics it is therefore important to eat a lot of live yoghurt and take a B complex supplement to restore your body's good bacteria quickly and prevent the fungi from moving in. Persistent fungal infections, if left unchecked, cause the production of antibody complexes, which can lead to a build-up of granulomas, which eventually calcify and could cause rheumatic-type pains in the joints.

PROGRESS IN COMBATING INFECTIOUS DISEASES

The eighteenth-century scientists Robert Hooke and Antony van Leeuwenhoek first opened the doors to the hidden world of microbes, but their 'little new animals' were merely acknowledged and observed using very simple microscopes.

These bacteria were thought to be the smallest living creatures until Martinus Beijerinck described 'a contagious living liquid' that caused tobacco mosaic disease in plants. It was not until the mid-twentieth century that this was found to contain infectious viral particles.

Medical progress in combating infectious diseases has been outstanding since the dawn of microbiology. Before this, epidemics of disease used to wipe out whole populations. During the Justinian era, plague killed two-thirds of the inhabitants of the major Roman cities. In fourteenth-century Europe, leprosy was a much-feared killer, as was the Plague, then known as the Black Death, which wiped out 25 million people in medieval times. Scarlet fever, measles and TB were the great fears in the nineteenth century, but we can now prevent, treat or cure all these diseases. AIDS may go down in history as the disease of the twentieth century, although cancer and heart disease, while not infectious, take more lives.

The battle against infectious diseases has, however, been fought in stages. In the late nineteenth century, Robert Koch, who was studying TB, came up with the 'germ theory' as a cause for these diseases. In the early twentieth century, Joseph Lister discovered antiseptics – prior to this, infections claimed the lives of many. His discovery brought vital developments in hygiene and public health, which continue to improve to this day.

Paul Erlich established the early basis for chemotherapy. Alexander Fleming's discovery of penicillin heralded the beginnings of modern antibiotics since used so successfully to wipe out bacterial infections. And Edward Jenner introduced vaccination, which provides resistance to specific diseases and is now widely used as a preventative measure.

Yet, in spite of these great leaps forward, the bugs are fighting back: they are changing and becoming resistant to our weapons. The search is on for alternative or new forms of treatment and prevention to combat these new or altered diseases. There are several ways forward: principally these involve finding further methods of killing or disarming the causative agents and stimulating the body's own defence mechanisms. Researchers are not only looking to the future, but also into past treatments used by ancient Greeks, Egyptians and Romans as well as present methods used by other cultures. Part 3 of this book follows some of the natural lines of inquiry.

....

CHAPTER 6

UNDERSTANDING AUTO-IMMUNITY

Auto-immunity is when the body's immune system attacks itself – possibly because it no longer recognises its own 'troops'. To understand this, we need to be familiar with the theory of how the immune system tells the difference between self and an invader (non-self).

DISTINGUISHING FRIEND FROM FOE

How do the defending white cells know what to attack and what to protect? The answer lies in the master computer, the thymus. Since before you were born it has been giving each of your cells an 'identity disc' and a code which is recorded in its 'memory banks'.

Think of your body as a country where every individual cell has been taught to speak the same language – English. You can immediately recognise someone from another country because they speak a different language. When your immune army recognises a foreigner, it immediately assumes that it is there to attack and so arrests the invader and destroys it.

There are three problems here:

1. The foreigner may not be hostile; it may even be trying to be helpful, e.g. a newly transplanted heart. In order to stop

an organ being recognised as an outsider, doctors therefore have to give the patient immune-suppressing drugs.

2. A French person could come into this country and speak such perfect English that we might not recognise them as foreign. A similar sort of situation occurs if a virus gets into your body and manages to enter one of your cells before it gets caught. The immune army recognises your cell, but not necessarily the invader within, and so it doesn't attack. Meanwhile, the virus takes over your cell's DNA and gets it to make its own instead so that your cell makes hundreds of new aliens! One of your cells, the cytotoxic T cell is programmed to recognise this trick. When it picks up 'two languages' it destroys the virus and the host cell, so it depends on luck or an efficient immune system as to whether or not the virus gets discovered in time.

3. The third loophole is the American who just happens to have English as his native language as well. All the immune cells recognise this cell as self and leave it alone. The bug which causes syphilis – *Treponema* – is like this. The antigen or 'identity disc' on its surface is the same as that on some of your heart muscle cells, cardiolipin. Treponema can therefore create havoc in the body for some time before it is checked. When the immune system eventually realises which traitor is doing the damage, it attacks it. But, in so doing, it also attacks the heart muscle which has the same code. These days it is possible to destroy *Treponema* but it is important to do so before the body has recognised it as foreign. Otherwise the immune system will carry on attacking the heart muscle even after the bug has been destroyed.

HOW ARE THE IDENTITY DISCS WRITTEN?

Our cells obviously neither speak nor write – the identity discs are therefore written with amino acids. A cell which carries a disc bearing English words like 'ship' or 'star' would be recognised as a skin, liver or whatever cell belonging to self and left alone by the immune army. Whereas cells carrying labels like 'foyq' or 'qdbg' would be destroyed. It is a very clever system but, as with all systems, there are some problems.

Firstly, if the body makes a simple spelling mistake and writes 'stau' instead of 'star' then the immune system will destroy the mislabelled cell. This wouldn't matter if it was an isolated error but if the body kept writing 'stau' then an auto-immune disease could follow, where our immune cells destroy our own body cells because the label is wrong.

Secondly, when the immune cells are overworked or understaffed, they may make a mistake and not recognise an 'English' word as English. In this case they would again attack our own cells in an auto-immune response.

HOW DO MISTAKES OCCUR?

Auto-immunity is, in effect, a language problem – misunderstandings due to errors in communication. It is surprising that there aren't more errors really. The average English-speaking person has around 100,000 words available to him/her and we're always making communication mistakes. The immune system can synthesise around 10 million!

Examples of auto-immune conditions are: pernicious and haemolytic anaemias, Addison's disease, systemic lupus erythematosis and rheumatoid arthritis. Ulcerative colitis is possibly caused by confusion between a marker on the colon (large intestine) and a bacterial inhabitant of the gut, E. coli. The immune cells therefore attack both, causing inflammation of the colon. Another interesting example is sperm. Because there is no sperm present at birth, it is not marked as 'self' and therefore kept separate from the immune cells. In a rare complication of mumps, it is possible for the virus to attack the separating membrane, so the immune cells fail to recognise the sperm as self and attack. Protein from the lens of the eye is similarly not recognised as self and so is protected from immune cells.

All your body's cells have their own identity, function and needs. To stay healthy, these individuals have to live together in harmony. Unfortunately there are many enemies which can upset this ideal state, from poor diet and lack of exercise to environmental pollution and stress. When things get out of control, errors can be made and civil war can break out. So look after your inner army – one day your health and life may depend on it.

CHAPTER 7

....

UNDERSTANDING AND ELIMINATING ALLERGIES

Allergy occurs when the body alters its normal immune response in some way, due to the presence of an allergen. Allergens are substances which bring about this immune response, and the odd thing about them is that they are not always harmful in themselves. Rather, it is the allergic individual who produces the wrong response. Interestingly, though, many allergy sufferers are immune-deficient in other ways too.

In the case of contact allergies, such as sensitivity to jewellery or detergents, it is the lymphocytes and macrophages which over-react, but in most other allergies it is the antibody response which is over-reactive. The role of antibodies in allergy was not well known until 1967, when the antibody IgE was discovered and associated with hayfever. IgE antibodies attach themselves to 'mast cells' in the body. When the offending allergen combines with its specific IgE antibody, the IgE molecule triggers the mast cell to release granules containing histamine and other chemicals that cause the symptoms of classic allergy – skin rashes, hayfever, rhinitis, sinusitis, asthma and eczema. Severe food allergies to, for example, shellfish or peanuts, cause immediate gastro-intestinal upsets or swelling in the face or throat. Such allergies are immediate, severe, inflammatory reactions. They can be life-threatening and require urgent medical attention.

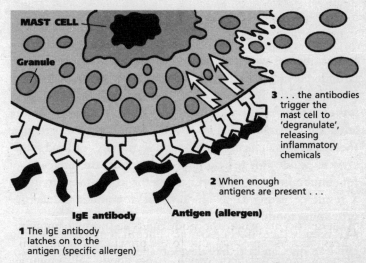

MAST CELL

Granule

3 . . . the antibodies trigger the mast cell to 'degranulate', releasing inflammatory chemicals

2 When enough antigens are present . . .

IgE antibody   **Antigen (allergen)**

1 The IgE antibody latches on to the antigen (specific allergen)

Figure 2 – How IgE-based Allergic Reactions Happen

DELAYED OR HIDDEN ALLERGIES

Not all reactions are immediate, nor do they all involve the IgE family of antibodies. The emerging view now is that most food allergies and intolerances (sometimes diplomatically called 'idiosyncratic' reactions) are not IgE based. There is a new school of thought that such intolerances involve another antibody – IgG – and possibly IgA. According to Dr James Braly, Medical Director of Immuno Laboratories:

> Food allergy is not rare, nor are the effects limited to the air passages, the skin and digestive tract. Most food allergies are delayed reactions, taking anywhere from an hour to three days to show themselves, and are therefore much harder to detect. Delayed food allergy appears to be simply the inability of your digestive tract to prevent

large quantities of partially digested and undigested food from entering the bloodstream.

IgG antibodies were first discovered in the 1960s and are still considered rather irrelevant by some conventional allergists. The problem, say the critics, is that the IgG antibodies may serve as 'tags' but don't initiate a reaction. However, say the advocates, a large build-up of IgG antibodies to a particular food indicates a chronic, long-term sensitivity, or food intolerance. While IgE reactions are immediate, the build-up of IgG antibodies may be a primary factor in food sensitivity, as a result of eating large amounts of a number of allergy-provoking foods.

Recently there has been some concern about giving young children nuts, in case they develop allergies to them later on. However, the nutrient value of nuts far outweighs any risk of sensitization, and, indeed, should help lessen susceptibility to allergies.

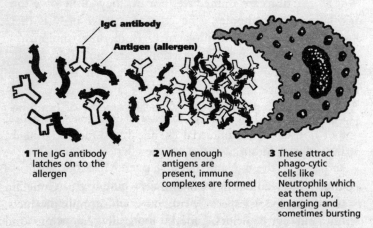

1 The IgG antibody latches on to the allergen

2 When enough antigens are present, immune complexes are formed

3 These attract phago-cytic cells like Neutrophils which eat them up, enlarging and sometimes bursting

Figure 3 – How IgG-based Allergic Reactions Happen

How IgG and IgE antibodies relate is another area of debate. Allergy specialist Dr James Braly has seen a number of patients who have both an immediate and delayed reaction to a food, suggesting a link between the immediate short-term IgE type reaction and the delayed IgG reaction.

WHAT CAUSES ALLERGIES?

Cases of allergies are rapidly increasing and are now thought to affect as many as one in three people. But it's not known whether this is due to an overall decline in our immunity, an increased burden on our immune system, or perhaps a bit of both.

Allergies can sometimes run in families: high total IgE levels can be inherited, as can faulty T cell response. The allergy, however, may not take the same form down the generations. Allergic symptoms also change with age. For example, a baby with eczema may grow out of it, only to become an adult who suffers from hayfever.

Common Allergens

Inhalant Dust and animal fur; moulds and perfumes; pollen; industrial, domestic or agricultural chemicals; gas; smoke; exhaust fumes; air conditioning or propellant gases.

Contact Nickel; jewellery; soaps and detergents; bleaches; other household or industrial chemicals; cosmetics; animals; paints; dyes; glues.

Other Bites and stings from insects; drugs, e.g. penicillin and aspirin; foods, especially fish, nuts, wheat, milk products, meat and eggs; artificial foods, especially colourings and flavourings.

COMMON ALLERGIC REACTIONS

These are usually grouped according to the areas they affect.

The Skin

Contact with an allergen can bring about various forms of dermatitis, hives and eczema.

Hives

Hives are large, whitish, raised areas on the skin, with an itching, red centre. They are often caused by a reaction to an insect bite or a contact allergen such as a plant. They sometimes come and go, in which case it is difficult to find the cause.

Eczema

This can be very itchy, and is usually worse in winter. It may then disappear completely or come and go, spreading to other areas. Wool can sometimes cause this or other types of skin reaction, but if the eczema persists there is nothing for it but to go through the whole list of possible allergens. It is helpful to think back to the day before each incident occurred, particularly the first one.

It is far better to trace the cause of the eczema and remove it if possible, rather than resort to cortisone creams or antihistamines (which are all immuno-suppressants), but this is not always practical. Food is often a cause of eczema, and food allergies are worth investigating.

The Head

Allergic symptoms may affect the eyes, nose, ears, lips or brain.

Migraine

Some forms of migraine can be caused by allergy, but it is not easy to find the cause; there are different triggers for different people. It seems that allergens may cause blood platelets clumps together thus slowing down the blood flow to the head.

There are whole lists of foods and chemicals which have been cited as potential triggers for migraine, the most common being cheese, chocolate, yeast, food flavours and colours, red wine, coffee, tea and sugar. Some medicines, like the Pill, and some household chemicals have also been implicated. Headaches may also be brought about by other factors, such as misalignment of the vertebrae or mineral deficiencies.

Hayfever

As well as causing running nose, sneezing and watery eyes, hayfever can also alter mood. Many sufferers, although by no means all, relieve their symptoms by switching to an unrefined diet low in wheat and sugar products. Hayfever can sometimes develop into bronchial asthma, slipping, so to speak, from the nose to the chest.

Asthma and other Conditions thought to be Allergy-Related

Asthma is not always due to allergy, but if the patient has previously suffered from eczema or hayfever, it is probably a contributory factor. Swelling occurs in the lining of the air tubes in the lung, and the muscle around the air tube contracts, possibly due to an imbalance of calcium and magnesium in the diet. An asthmatic thus usually needs more dietary magnesium, as this is deficient in the average Western diet. Asthmatics are also sensitive to metabisulphite (the preservative in wine and squashes) and the orange colouring tartrazine, as well as to some drugs.

Allergic symptoms may also affect other areas of the body, such as the hands, stomach, feet, blood vessels and bladder. With most allergic problems, it is a question of trying to find the triggers that bring about the condition. To complicate matters, there are often several triggers, not just one, which makes them not only difficult to find but also difficult to eliminate from our diet or immediate environment.

Behavioural Problems

Hyperactivity, vandalism and crime are going up all over the world and not just in proportion to the increase in population. Quite a few studies now show a link between diet and such anti-social behaviour. It appears that unreal fears and phobias may also be associated with food or chemical sensitivity. Work has been done with prisoners and juvenile offenders which has shown that dietary changes can reduce aggressive and destructive behaviour. Animals put on a diet where the natural food has been replaced by highly processed foodstuffs have consistently shown increased aggressive behaviour.

Alcoholism

Studies done with alcoholics now show that people often have sensitivities to wheat, corn, rye, malt, sugar or yeast. People without sensitivities to these foods are less likely to become addicted to alcohol, even though they may drink a lot more than those who are.

Fits and Heart Problems

Ingestion of or exposure to food or chemical allergens can bring on fits, irregular heartbeats, high blood pressure, chest pains and blood clots. Research is still relatively new and incomplete in this area, but it is possible that some strokes and heart-related problems could be avoided if only we could recognise our food and chemical sensitivities, deficiencies and excesses.

Inflammatory Bowel Diseases

Conditions such as Crohn's disease and ulcerative colitis are often blamed on food sensitivities, but exclusion diets should not be undertaken without professional guidance, as people with gut problems are often already very nutrient-deficient due to the inability of the gut to digest and absorb normally. Antibodies to cow's milk and salicylates are often found in people with ulcerative colitis, but avoiding foods containing these does not always bring relief. Supplements (of zinc, in particular) are often helpful.

Arthritis

Food and chemical allergies have been cited as major factors in worsening symptoms of rheumatoid arthritis. There have been remarkable claims from people confined to wheelchairs whose symptoms improved, to the extent that they were able to get up and walk, after eliminating certain foods like red meat or perhaps dairy products, wheat, tea or coffee from their diet. These foods have also been labelled as aggravators in cases of osteo-arthritis. It should be mentioned that it is usually one or two of these major risk foods that are a problem and they vary from person to person.

ALLERGY TESTS – ARE THEY WORTH IT?

Testing for allergy is notoriously difficult. There are numerous allergy tests available, each claiming to be accurate. But trials have shown that such tests can produce widely varying results. Some are, however, reasonably accurate, especially in detecting particular types of allergies.

Skin Prick Testing

A drop of allergen is put on the skin, which is scratched to allow the allergen to enter the body. Inflammation indicates a positive response. This is a good test for skin-related allergies but not so accurate for inhalant or food allergies.

Rast

For the RAST (Radio Allergo Sorbent Test), serum is separated from a blood sample and placed on samples of allergens. If the serum contains IgE to that allergen, a complex is formed. The level of sensitivity can also be measured. This is the most accurate test for IgE based reactions and more likely to pick up food allergies than skin tests, as long as the food allergies are IgE based.

IgG ELISA

The ELISA (Enzyme Linked Immuno Sorbent Assay) Test also uses blood serum to test reactions to various allergens, and can test for IgG positivity and levels of sensitivity. This method has proved to be highly accurate for IgG detection.

Avoidance Testing

Perhaps one of the most accurate ways for an individual to discover allergens is to avoid suspect foods for a time and then watch for any reaction when they are reintroduced into the diet. Foods that provoke an immediate IgE-type response may have to be avoided for life. Others that produce a more delayed, IgG reaction may be reduced or avoided for some time. It is generally recommended that you avoid suspect foods for at least a month, then test. After long-term avoidance (up to six months) it is unlikely that any 'memory' of a reaction to that food will remain. Another option, after a strict, one-month avoidance, is to 'rotate' foods so an IgG sensitive food is only eaten every four days, to reduce the build-up of allergen-antibody complexes.

Should you wish to investigate having your allergies tested, we recommend that you see a nutrition consultant (see Useful Addresses) who can advise you on which kind of test is most appropriate for you.

PART 3

SIX STEPS TO IMMUNE POWER

CHAPTER 8

IMMUNE-BOOSTING FOODS

When you think about it, nature has set up the perfect system: it provides foods in seasonal rotation so that we do not become sensitive to them, and foods packed with immune power boosters in late summer and autumn to prepare us for the winter ahead when the cold and flu bugs reach their peak. All vegetable matter can be recycled, either by passing through animals or by rotting, thus releasing vital minerals back into the soil and then back into the food supply (unless we put our vegetable rubbish in non-degradable plastic bags in the dustbin, of course).

The trouble is that man thinks he knows better than nature. Seasonal food is now available all year round, either preserved or imported. Food can now be stored for so long that few, if any, vitamins remain. Nutrients are often processed out of food in order to increase its shelf-life and keep it free from bugs; after all, no self-respecting weevil would want to eat nutrient-deficient food. We spray pesticides on our food to stop other creatures from eating our precious stores, even though they are poisons which have some effect on us too. Virtually anything added to food is aimed at improving its shelf-life or appearance rather than its nutritional value. Our bodies steadily accumulate stores of toxins, like lead, mercury, aluminium and cadmium, all to the detriment of our health.

The food we eat affects our thoughts, behaviour, mood and

temper, as well as our ability to exercise, relax and sleep. It alters our hormones, skin, blood, organs, bones and muscles. And it has an impact on our immune system. Food provides the building blocks of the body; refined, processed, nutrient-deficient foods give us inferior building blocks. We may be able to build a large house, especially if we eat a lot of them, but how strong is it? Will it stand the test of time or will it only take a little wolf to huff and puff and expose our unhealthy bacon?

RECIPE FOR A STRONG IMMUNE SYSTEM

We use food to make every part of our immune system, so its strength depends on the quality of our food. To help build a strong immune system:

• Of the total calorific intake, 60 per cent is best taken in the form of carbohydrate. This should be mainly wholefoods, including grains other than wheat (our national addiction), along with plenty of fruit and vegetables.

• Not much more than around 20 per cent of our calories should come from fat, and most of that should be the essential fatty acids found in nuts, seeds and fish.

• The remaining 20 per cent of our calories should provide all the amino acids which make up good-quality protein.

PROTEINS

Surprisingly, there are quite a few people who are deficient in protein, even in developed countries which appear to have ample food. If you answer 'yes' to a lot of the questions over-leaf, you could be too. People most at risk are those on imbalanced slimming diets, vegans or vegetarians who don't learn about amino acid combining, fast-food addicts, people who live alone, and children. Children and young people need a lot of protein for growth but many choose a low-nutrient, fast-food diet. Some become vegetarian when their parents are not, and so tend to be given the same meals, but without the meat.

Are You Protein-Deficient?

1. Do you find it difficult to hold yourself up straight when sitting or standing?
2. Do you have rounded shoulders, a sunken chest or flat feet?
3. Do your hair and nails grow slowly?
4. Is your memory slipping or do you have difficulty concentrating?
5. Do you get mood swings – depression, anxiety and irritability?
6. Do you have difficulty sleeping?
7. Do you get frequent infections?
8. Do you get muscle aches and pains?
9. Do you feel that you look older than you are?
10. Do you constantly feel hungry?
11. Do you have weight problems?
12. Do you get indigestion or constipation?
13. Do you have very low blood pressure?
14. Do you suffer from water retention?

What are Proteins?

Protein is the basic constituent of all living cells. Three-quarters of the dry weight of most body cells is protein. Proteins make up hormones, enzymes, neurotransmitters, immune cells and antibodies. The name comes from Proteus, a mythological figure who, like protein, could change his form. If we eat beef protein or bean protein, we break it down into its constituent amino acids and then make it up again into the protein we require. The amino acids themselves perform essential functions. Some control memory, sleep, moods, energy levels, relaxation, tension and how our immune systems respond.

Roughly every seven years we have a new body. This is, of course, an over-simplification, as brain cells are replaced very slowly if at all, while, at the other end of the scale, we get a new skin every three or four weeks and two new gut linings a week. Every second, we create thousands of new immune cells and antibody molecules. Our spares and repairs department needs an awful lot of amino acid building blocks.

The Amino Acids

Amino acids are the constituents of protein – there are eight that are vital to life and they are found in meat, fish and dairy produce, as well as beans, lentils, nuts and other 'seed' foods. The 'friendly' bacteria that live in our gut, performing some important jobs, make very small amounts for us all the time, and, without this background level, we would suffer from severe mood swings.

The essential amino acids mostly lacking in plants are methionine, tryptophan and lysine. The first, methionine, is essential for pregnant women because it is required for the development of a baby's thymus, a major part of the immune system. Soya beans and legumes are a poor source of methionine. And grains are deficient in lysine. However, if you combine a grain (such as rice) with a legume (such as lentils), you get a much better balance of amino acids and hence more usable protein. Tryptophan-rich foods include fish, turkey, chicken, cottage cheese, avocados, bananas and wheatgerm.

Amino acids are the 'alphabet' of the body. Each of the body's cells is labelled with an arrangement of amino acids.

This is read by the body's immune system, enabling it to recognise friend or foe, and by the ribosomes which make all the proteins necessary for the body to grow, repair itself and reproduce. Amino acids make up the chemical of life, our DNA. Antibodies, too, are protein, and lymphocytes have a high requirement for amino acids for their production and function. The amino acids which stimulate the immune system most are alanine, aspartic acid, cysteine, glycine, lysine, methionine, glutamine and threonine. Those used for detoxification include glycine, methionine, cysteine, glutamine, taurine and tyrosine.

If food is eaten whole and unrefined, complete with the nutrients required for its utilisation, we obtain enough of these amino acids. An imbalanced diet, however, can easily create an imbalance in the body's amino acid pool, which is not so easy to sort out. It is therefore important to have a full range of amino acids in our diet, but here we list a few which apply specifically to the immune system.

Methionine

In experiments, scientists have tried to recreate what they thought was Earth's primitive atmosphere, containing just carbon, hydrogen, nitrogen, oxygen and sulphur. These are the components of methionine, probably the oldest amino acid. Good dietary sources are meat, fish, cheese, eggs, nuts and seeds (especially sunflower), wheatgerm, wholegrains and quinoa (a grain which cooks like rice).

Methionine can relieve pain because it is a component of various endorphins (chemicals involved in killing pain and producing feelings of well-being). It is essential for the development of the foetal immune system and for the immune systems of children. This is important to note in the case of children on soya diets or soya-based infant formulae who take no milk or meat, as soya is very deficient in methionine. Methionine deficiency might not be noticed until the baby grows into a more sickly child. So children and pregnant mothers, in particular, need foods sufficient in methionine.

Cysteine and Glutathione

Cysteine is very important for the immune system, mainly because it is turned into glutathione in the body, which is highly concentrated in the thymus gland.

Glutathione also protects us from toxins. We are exposed to a lot of toxic substances in air, food and water. Provided there is sufficient cysteine present, the body can increase its levels of glutathione to detoxify, for example, alcohol, exhaust fumes, pesticides and carcinogens within the body. High cysteine levels are associated with health, longevity and a reduced risk of cancer. In chronic infections, such as AIDS, one of the major concerns is a depletion of glutathione.

Glutathione is an antioxidant and helps protect us against toxic forms of oxygen, especially those resulting from damaged fats in fried food. It is, in fact, such a primitive and universal antioxidant that scientists have even considered adding it to dying lakes to restore life. Glutathione is vital for macrophages to make the chemicals they need to kill invaders, for lymphocyte production and for red blood cell membranes.

It works with anthocyans, a powerful group of antioxidants found in vegetables, fruits and berries (especially grapes and bilberries), which have the power to recycle glutathione. For this reason, supplementing 'reduced glutathione', together with a source of anthocyans, is a very effective way to improve immune function. Glutathione supplements must be coated, otherwise the gluathione can break down in the stomach. An alternative strategy is to ensure adequate cysteine in your diet. This, too, can be supplemented as N-acetyl-cysteine (NAC). The best foods for cysteine are meat, eggs, soya, quinoa, seeds, nuts, onions and garlic.

Glutamine

Glutamine is another amino acid critical for the immune system. It is semi-essential, which means that the body can make it but functions better if we take some in via our food. Glutamine is needed for immune cells to multiply and mature and helps them stay fighting fit. During infections and traumas, such as surgery or burns, glutamine gets used up at a rapid rate. Taking in more of this amino acid helps to boost the body's immune response. For this reason it is now given to burn victims and others who experience immuno-suppression, such as those with AIDS and auto-immune diseases. It can also be used to make glutathione.

There is no easy way to substantially increase your glutamine intake from food, unless you happen to like raw meat, fish or eggs (glutamine is especially rich in muscle and rapidly denatured by cooking). Eating sushi (Japanese raw fish) frequently is about the only way you can substantially up your glutamine intake. Glutamine can, however, be supplemented as a tasteless powder. A heaped teaspoon (5g) a day can make a difference to the immune system, while, in severe immuno-suppression, such as AIDS, up to 40g a day may be needed for maximum benefit.

Getting the Right Balance of Amino Acids

Correct amino acid balance is necessary for many things in the body – good posture, strong muscles, reproduction, growth, body repair, healthy hair, healthy nails, and so on. But for the immune system, proteins, and hence amino acids – in their right balance, are essential to make immune cells and antibodies to combat infection.

Many people find that, when their amino acid balance is restored, they no longer crave junk foods. Of course, it is perfectly possible to live healthily and well on a vegetarian or vegan diet, although people who do so should make sure that they know how to combine foods to increase the balance of amino acids they are receiving. For example, by eating grains, such as rice, with lentils, beans or tofu, you improve the balance of amino acids and increase the usability of the protein these foods contain. Part 5 of this book explains what you need to eat to get the right balance of amino acids.

CARBOHYDRATES

Carbohydrates make up the greater part of our diet and are obtained from grains, fruit, vegetables, legumes, nuts and most processed foods. They are broken down in the body into simple sugars, which are used to make energy.

Complex carbohydrates, i.e. unrefined foods, are much the best way to obtain these, as they come complete with the nutrients necessary for their utilisation. They are a bit like time-release capsules. Simple sugars and refined carbohydrates flood the system with sugars as soon as they are absorbed, providing a quick flash of energy, followed by a long period of lethargy. In contrast, complex carbohydrates release their sugars slowly so that the level of sugar in the blood remains roughly within a normal range, instead of going up and down like a see-saw. When it is low, we crave sweets and become easily irritated, moody and uncooperative. Whereas, if we eat sufficient and appropriate food, we feel fine, think quickly and clearly, lose our hunger pangs and even find sweets distasteful.

Starch

Starch is the fundamental complex carbohydrate that we consume in grains, bread, pulses and starchy vegetables like potatoes. Although we appear to have a wide variety of foods to choose from, most of us seem to be addicted to wheat. Pasta, pizzas, pastries, biscuits, pies, bread, cakes and many breakfast cereals are apparently different foods, but in reality are all wheat. As a consequence of this monotonous diet, and the difficulty the body has in digesting gluten (the protein in wheat), it is one of the most common allergy-provoking foods. If you eat less wheat and vary your choice of grain, your immune system has an easier time. Have barley, oats, rye, rice, corn (maize), buckwheat and millet instead. Choose wholegrain breakfast cereals rather than sugar- and salt-laden, refined ones, and eat lots of vegetables, both raw and cooked. Try oat or millet flakes for breakfast (cold or as porridge), Scandinavian-style rye bread, buckwheat spaghetti, sugar-free corn flakes, brown rice or barley with your meal.

It is a good habit to eat a few raw vegetables as a starter before a cooked meal. This helps your immune system to deal with the following food without having such a fight. It used to be thought that digestive leucocytosis (which involves white blood cells migrating to the gut wall to be on alert, and their subsequent destruction) occurred whatever we ate. But it has now been found that it only happens when we eat cooked food. Raw food does not waste immune soldiers, so, eaten before a cooked meal, it lessens the overall destruction of white blood cells.

Sugars

We need sugars or, more precisely, glucose, which is the final breakdown product of all carbohydrate, because it is the major fuel for the brain, muscles and the immune system. But sugars have got a bad name, mainly because our intake is again out of balance with our needs. At present, one-third of the carbohydrate intake in the Western world is in the form of sucrose (refined sugar). This 'food' provides nothing except energy, and gets stored as saturated fat if it is not used. Much of it is hidden in highly processed foods and drinks, invisible but destructive. This is because sucrose is not only nutrient-free – it actually requires nutrients for its metabolism so it has to steal them from somewhere else. This is one of the reasons why vitamin B deficiency is so common – we waste precious nutrients, including the B vitamins, trying to process this useless sugar.

FIBRE

There are many types of fibre. Gums, resins and pectins (found in apples and bananas), as well as cellulose (the major component of plant cell walls), all provide fibre. Ruminant animals can break cellulose down into sugar, but we cannot do this. However, the 'friendly' bugs in our gut do need cellulose in order to stay healthy. So eating wholefoods and greens keeps our welcome guests happy and, in return, they keep us clean inside and provide us with a bonus of B vitamins, essential amino acids and fats. What a bargain!

A clean digestive tract is also obviously better for the immune system. If we are repeatedly constipated, there is a build-up of toxins which can be absorbed into the bloodstream. The immune system has to deal with this and no self-respecting bacteria wants to live in a constipated colon. They move out and make room for the less reputable varieties, like Candida, who are willing to slum it in these unhealthy living conditions.

LIPIDS

There are two types of lipids, fats and oils. Lipids are very important, as they help to form the membrane that surrounds every single cell in the body. With the right sort of lipids, cell membranes are strong; without them, they are weak and more prone to attack. Lipids are also an important component of brain and nervous tissue which contain large amounts of 'phospholipids', such as phosphatidyl choline (PC) and phosphatidyl serine (PS).

'Bad' Fats

In Britain we eat, on average, 125g of fat a day, which is 42 per cent of our calorie intake. We are advised to reduce this to 100g or less (the equivalent of 25–30 per cent of our calorie intake). Not only do we tend to eat too much fat in general, but we also usually eat too much of the fats that are not so good for us.

Saturated fats, mainly from meat and dairy produce, are not essential for the body; high intakes have been linked to heart disease, bowel cancer and many other problems. Yet most of the fats we eat are saturated, mainly of animal origin.

Other lipids which do us no good at all, and in fact harm us, are processed, heated polyunsaturates. This is because polyunsaturates are more prone to oxidation, which, over time, can wreak havoc in our bodies. So frying foods in polyunsaturated oil, such as sunflower oil, is very detrimental to our health.

Good Lipids

Some lipids are quite happily assimilated by the body, while others are absolutely necessary for good health – without them we simply would not be able to function. The former include monounsaturated fats such as olive oil. Polyunsaturated oils – in their unrefined, unheated form – are associated with a decreased risk of heart disease, stronger immune system, better skin and much more. If they are heated, however, these properties are cancelled out and they actually increase the risk of cancer as well as other problems.

Arachidonic acid is a fatty acid found in meat and dairy produce, so it is not usually lacking in people's diets. It is necessary for several reactions in the body, including creating inflammation and helping blood clot. Too much, however, can cause these reactions in excess, exacerbating conditions such as heart disease and arthritis. It is not essential to get arachidonic acid in our diets as our bodies can make it from other fats (see below).

Essential Fatty Acids

To further complicate the issue, some kinds of polyunsaturated fats provide essential fatty acids which are needed by the body but cannot be made or converted from existing fats, so we have to get them from our diets. These are essential for good immune function, blood clotting, nerve impulses, brain function, digestion, transport of cholesterol and the strength of cell membranes. The important ones are linoleic acid, belonging to the Omega 6 group of fatty acids, and alpha-linolenic acid, belonging to the Omega 3 group.

The Omega 6 Family

The grandmother of the Omega 6 family is linoleic acid. This is converted by the body into gamma-linolenic acid (GLA), provided you have enough vitamin B6, biotin, zinc and magnesium to drive the enzyme that makes the conversion. Evening primrose oil and borage oil are the richest known sources of GLA and, by supplementing these direct, you need take in less overall oil to get an optimal intake of Omega 6 oils. The ideal intake is probably around 150mg of GLA a day, which is equivalent to 1500mg of evening primrose oil, or 750mg of high-potency borage oil.

GLA then gets converted into DGLA and from there into prostaglandins which are extremely active hormone-like substances in the body. The particular kind of prostaglandins made from these Omega 6 oils are called 'Series 1 prostaglandins' (PG1s).

PG1s are involved in the regulation of the T-suppressor cells (crucial for immune function) and also reduce the stickiness of blood, thereby decreasing the risk of heart disease.

They keep the blood thin, relax the blood vessels, lower blood pressure, help maintain water balance in the body, decrease inflammation and pain, improve nerve and immune function, and help insulin to work (which is good for blood sugar balance). This is only a short list. As each year passes, more and more health-promoting functions are being found. Prostaglandins themselves cannot be supplemented, as they are very short-lived. Instead we rely on a good intake of Omega 6 oils, from which the body can make the prostaglandins we need.

The body can also convert Omega 6 oils into arachidonic acid, which goes on to form 'Series 2 prostaglandins' (PG2s), which include a sub-group called the leukotrienes (known to increase inflammation and blood clotting). Although these are sometimes essential, an excess of such activity can be harmful.

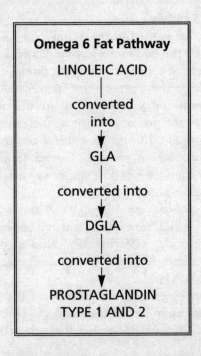

Omega 6 Fat Pathway

LINOLEIC ACID

|

converted
into

↓

GLA

|

converted into

↓

DGLA

|

converted into

↓

PROSTAGLANDIN
TYPE 1 AND 2

Furthermore, the leukotrienes are involved in asthma and other allergic conditions. PG2s are derived mainly from meat and dairy produce, although small amounts come from seeds.

Omega 6 oils come exclusively from seeds and their oils. The best seed oils are hemp, pumpkin, sunflower, safflower, sesame, corn, walnut, soybean and wheatgerm oil. About half the fats in these oils comes from the Omega 6 family, mainly as linoleic acid. An optimal intake would be 1 tablespoon of oil a day, or 1 heaped tablespoon of ground seeds.

The Omega 3 Family

The modern diet is likely to be more deficient in Omega 3 oils than Omega 6s simply because the grandmother of the Omega 3 family, alpha–linolenic acid, and her metabolically active grandchildren, eicosapentaenoic acid (EPA) and docosahexaenoic acid (DHA), are more prone to damage in cooking and food processing. You can see this increasing complexity as we move up the food chain. For example,

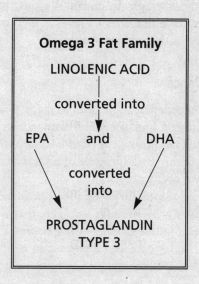

Omega 3 Fat Family

LINOLENIC ACID

converted into

EPA   and   DHA

converted
into

PROSTAGLANDIN
TYPE 3

plankton, the staple food of small fish, is rich in alpha-linolenic acid. The conversion is continued as they are eaten by carnivorous fish (mackerel and herring) which, in turn, are eaten by seals which have the highest EPA and DHA concentration. This is why Eskimos, who eat seals, benefit from a ready-made meal of EPA and DHA.

In the body, these lipids are converted into 'Series 3 prostaglandins' (PG3s). These are essential for immune function, reducing inflammation, reducing the stickiness of blood, proper brain function, vision, learning ability, co-ordination and mood, as well as controlling blood cholesterol and fat levels, metabolism, and maintaining water balance.

The best seed oils for Omega 3 oils are flax (also known as linseed), hemp and pumpkin. In much the same way as evening primrose oil bypasses the first 'conversion' stage of linoleic acid, eating carnivorous fish or their oils bypasses the first two conversion stages of alpha-linolenic acid to provide EPA and DHA. This is why fish-eaters like the Japanese have a level of Omega 3 oils in their body fat which is three times higher than the average American. Vegans, who eat more seeds and nuts, have an Omega 3 level in their body fat which is twice as high as the average American.

Essential Balance

Most people are deficient in both Omega 6 and Omega 3 lipids. In addition, a high intake of saturated fats and damaged polyunsaturated fats (known as trans fats) stops the body making good use of the small quantity of essential fats the average person eats in a day.

It is therefore important to balance our intake of the various essential fatty acids in order to ensure that we have a beneficial balance of prostaglandins in our bodies. For example, a deficiency of PG1s tends to be present in people with auto-immune diseases like rheumatoid arthritis, as well as in those with multiple sclerosis; this is thought to be due to the effect these PGs have on the T-suppressor cells.

Ideally our diet should have high levels of both Omega 3 and 6 lipids. Differing views exist about the ideal ratio. The estimated intakes of our hunter–gatherer ancestors suggest that we need equal amounts, although some researchers advise twice as much Omega 6 as Omega 3 to match our relative need. Either way, the average diet is deficient in both, with excess Omega 6 in relation to Omega 3 fat.

Hemp seed oil from the cannabis plant is a good source of both types of lipids. Although it is illegal to grow the plant in many parts of the world, the seeds and fibre are legal. Hemp is now making a comeback, both as a source of nutrition, and as a fabric for clothes. Hemp seed oil is 19 per cent alpha-linolenic acid (Omega 3), 57 per cent linoleic acid and 2 per cent GLA (both Omega 6). It is the only common seed oil that provides significant amounts of all these essential fatty acid needs.

You can also buy organic seed oil blends, balanced for Omega 3 and Omega 6 oils, from health food stores. One such oil blend is Essential Balance (see Useful Addresses).

Alternatively, you can combine seeds. Sunflower and sesame are good sources of Omega 6; pumpkin provides reasonable quantities of both; and flax seed is richest in Omega 3. Put 1 measure each of sesame, sunflower and pumpkin seeds and 2 measures of flax seeds in a sealed jar in the fridge, away from light, heat and oxygen. Simply grind a handful and add 2 heaped tablespoons to your breakfast each morning to guarantee a good daily intake of essential fatty acids. Alternatively, add 1 spoonful and make up the difference with a salad dressing, nuts or seeds later in the day.

Because the oil in these seeds is unsaturated and prone to damage, it's important to buy fresh seeds that have been properly stored, with minimal exposure to heat, light and oxygen.

Omega 3	Omega 6
2.5–5 per cent of total calories 8–17g a day	3–5 per cent of total calories 10–17g a day
Hemp seed oil – 1 tablespoon or	Hemp seed oil – 1 tablespoon or
Flax seed oil – 1 tablespoon or	Evening primrose oil – 1000mg or
Flax seeds – 2 tablespoons or	Borage oil – 500mg or
EPA/DHA – 1000mg or	Sunflower seeds – 1 tablespoon or
Pumpkin seeds – 4 tablespoons or	Pumpkin seeds – 2 tablespoons or
A serving of carnivorous fish (e.g. tuna, mackerel, salmon, etc)	Sesame seeds – 1.5 tablespoons

Ideally, consume one item in each column per day to achieve your optimum intake of essential fatty acids. Individual needs do vary, however, so this is only a rough guide.

THE IMMUNE POWER DIET

Putting all this into practice in your diet is, without doubt, a powerful way to support your immune system. Part 5 of this book clearly explains what this means in terms of what you eat. However the general principles are as follows:

■ Have two servings of beans, lentils, quinoa (a grain that cooks like rice), tofu (soya), or 'seed' vegetables a day for protein, or one serving of fish or free-range chicken. Include both grains and beans/lentils in your daily diet to increase protein quality if you are vegetarian.

■ Eat plenty of complex carbohydrates, such as brown rice, millet, rye, oats, wholewheat, corn, quinoa, as cereal, breads or pasta. Avoid any form of sugar, and white, refined or processed food.

■ Have five servings of fresh fruit and vegetables each day, such as apples, pears, bananas, berries, melon or citrus fruit, and a mixture of dark green, leafy and root vegetables, such as watercress, carrots, sweet potatoes, broccoli, spinach, green beans, peas and peppers.

- Eat at least 1 heaped tablespoon of ground seeds or 1 tablespoon of cold-pressed seed oil a day. Avoid fried, burnt or browned food, hydrogenated fat and excess animal fat.

- Eat whole, organic, raw food as much as you can and drink about six glasses of water, diluted juices, herb or fruit teas each day.

CHAPTER 9

IMMUNE-BOOSTING NUTRIENTS

While you need up to 50g of protein a day, you need only a millionth of that amount, 50 micrograms, of selenium – a quantity too small to see. Yet, without micronutrients like selenium, your immune system won't work properly. Let's take a look at the key immune-boosting vitamins and minerals. Suggested doses are listed in the chart on page 161.

VITAMIN A

This is known as the growth vitamin, because it is necessary for the production of growth hormone, which in turn is responsible, not only for growth, but for maintaining an active thymus and hence a strong immune system. T cells are depleted if growth hormone is in short supply, as the thymus shrinks, becoming less active and less efficient at maturing T cells. B cells are also adversely affected.

Vitamin A is a powerful anti-viral vitamin, mainly because its inclusion in cell walls makes them stronger and more resistant to viral attack. It is particularly important for areas with a high risk of infection, such as the respiratory system, the gut and the genito-urinary tract. Body secretions, like sweat, tears and saliva, as well as the immune system's cells, all need vitamin A for the production of lysozyme, a protective anti-bacterial enzyme. People who regularly suffer from conjunctivitis are probably deficient in vitamin A (as well as vitamin C).

Which Foods are Best for Vitamin A (Retinol Beta-Carotene)?

Foods are listed in order of those that contain the most beta-carotene per calorie of food. The figures in brackets are the amount of retinol or beta-carotene in 100g, which is roughly equivalent to a cup or serving.

Beef liver	(35,778iu)	Broccoli	(1541iu)
Carrots	(28,125iu)	Apricots (fresh)	(2612iu)
Watercress	(4700iu)	Papayas	(2014iu)
Cabbage	(3000iu)	Asparagus	(829iu)
Squash	(7000iu)	Apricots (dried)	(7240iu)
Sweet potatoes	(17,055iu)	Peppers	(530iu)
Melon	(3224iu)	Tangerines	(920iu)
Pumpkin	(1600iu)	Nectarines	(730iu)
Mangoes	(3894iu)	Peaches	(535iu)
Tomatoes	(1133iu)	Watermelon	(365iu)

Both vitamin A and its precursor, beta-carotene, provide protection from cancer. You need more when you are fighting an infection (especially viral), if you smoke, if you are exposed to pollution, or if you are under considerable stress. It also helps heal many skin conditions, from acne to eczema.

Are You Deficient in Vitamin A?

The first signs of vitamin A deficiency are skin complaints such as dry, flaky skin, dandruff and acne. Frequent infections, cystitis or diarrhoea are another indication. Other symptoms include frequent mouth ulcers and poor night vision. In more pronounced vitamin A deficiency, children's growth rates slow down and eyes become dry and irritated. In severe deficiency, cataracts (and hence blindness) develop.

Vitamin A Supplements

When supplements of vitamin A are needed, they are best taken in the form of beta-carotene, as this form is not toxic and is only made into vitamin A as the body requires it. Diabetics are better advised to supplement vitamin A or cod liver oil, as they cannot convert beta-carotene into vitamin A. Supplements need to be taken with vitamin E to be most effective, as they protect each other.

B COMPLEX

This family of essential nutrients is important for every single cell of our bodies, including those of the immune system. Folic acid and pyridoxine (B6) probably have the most effect on immune function. Folic acid is essential for pregnant mothers and for the development of mature organs in the foetus. It has been found that a baby's thymus is larger and its immune system stronger if the mother has had a good supply of folic acid, choline, B12 and methionine. During pregnancy, folic acid is also necessary for all cell division, and therefore important for healing.

A B6 deficiency lessens the activity of the phagocytic cells so that they cannot clean up inside us as effectively as they should (remember, phagocytes get rid of 'invaders', dead cells and any other unwanted matter). B6 also helps the body make cysteine from methionine, a key amino acid for immunity.

Pantothenic acid (B5) is another immune stimulant, necessary for antibody production, helping macrophages and natural killer cells to do their job. The semi-essential nutrient choline, which used to be thought of as another B vitamin, is converted into a substance which increases lymphocyte production.

Which Foods are Best for B Vitamins?

Major sources of all B vitamins are liver, yeast, blackstrap molasses, and wholegrains, especially wheatgerm and rice bran. For specific B vitamins, see the following list:

- B1: Lamb, asparagus, mushrooms, peas, beans, watercress, lettuce, peppers

- B2: Broccoli, wheatgerm, milk, asparagus, mushrooms, watercress, cabbage

- B3: Tuna, chicken, lamb, wholewheat, courgettes, asparagus

- Folic acid: Wheatgerm, spinach, peanuts, sprouted seeds and beans, asparagus, broccoli

- B5: Mushrooms, lentils, eggs, avocado, wholewheat, alfalfa, peas, tomatoes

- B6: Kidney beans, cauliflower, Brussels sprouts, seeds and nuts

- B12: Oysters, sardines, tuna, meat, eggs, dairy produce

- Biotin: Almonds, cauliflower, corn, oysters, eggs

There are so many circumstances in which we need more B vitamins. Since bacteria in the digestive tract make some B vitamins, we need to take in more after a course of antibiotics which kill off many of these good bacteria. Anyone who is highly stressed, or takes a lot of sugar, alcohol or refined food, robs themselves of B vitamins. Be careful, however, about supplementing extra if you know you have a bacterial infection, as bacteria also need B vitamins.

Are You Deficient in B Vitamins?

The B vitamins are used by just about every cell in the body. Deficiency symptoms are therefore very varied, although there are almost always mental effects such as depression, anxiety, moodiness and difficulty with concentration. Energy is often low because B vitamins are needed to make energy from food. A host of other symptoms may also appear – like headaches, premenstrual tension, bad breath, dandruff, eczema, water retention, weight problems, sensitivity to light and so on.

Probably one of the most reliable physical guides to severe B vitamin deficiency is the mouth, and in particular the tongue (change in size, deep fissures, very smooth and sore, coating or off-colour), or cracked, sore lips and mouth corners. The obvious deficiency in the mouth will be extended to other areas of digestion, showing up as excessive gas and indigestion.

Vitamin B supplements

When supplementing B vitamins it is best to take a B complex, which gives a good balance of them all. Sometimes a single B vitamin is supplemented for a short time to restore a balance, but it should be taken with a low dose B complex or with plenty of B-rich food. A good B complex supplement provides somewhere between 25 and 75mg of B1, B2, B3, B5 and B6, plus 10mcg of B12, and 100mcg or more of folic acid and biotin.

VITAMIN C

In truth a whole book could be written about vitamin C and its effects on the immune system. There is no question that more vitamin C means better immune function. Here are some of its key roles in boosting your immunity:

- Vitamin C is strongly anti-viral. Many viruses, such as flu and the common cold, do not necessarily enter the bloodstream; rather, they spread in the mucus on the respiratory tract membranes. Consequently there is very little antibody stimulation and the job of defence falls to the T cells. Vitamin C has proved successful against every virus tested so far, from HIV to the common cold.[1]

- Prostaglandin production in blood platelets is boosted by vitamin C, in turn increasing T cell production.

- Vitamin C is needed for a special kind of cell division which results in a rapid increase of both B and T cells. The flu virus actually works by depressing this type of cell division.

- Infected cells produce more interferon when they have sufficient vitamin C. The vitamin C also blocks the synthesis of viral proteins which are essential for the infected cells to be replicated.

- Vitamin C can be bacteriostatic or bactericidal (i.e. it can hinder their growth or kill them, depending on the bug).

- C3 complement production is improved with vitamin C, which in turn triggers B cells to manufacture more antibodies, especially IgA, IgG and IgM.

- It stimulates non-lysozyme antibacterial factor (NLAF) found in tears. This is of particular importance for people who often suffer from eye infections.

- Vitamin C enables phagocytic cells to carry out their clearing-up function. They can only work if they contain at least 20mcg of vitamin C per 100 million cells.

- Vitamin C detoxifies, partially at least, many bacterial toxins (which often cause all the unpleasant symptoms), depending on the bug.

- Apart from stimulating natural anti-bacterial factors in the body, vitamin C also improves the performance of antibiotics.

- Mononuclear phagocytes, a special type of white blood cell, use vitamin C with hydrogen peroxide and some minerals, especially zinc compounds, to kill the invaders that they have captured. In those who are vitamin C deficient, bacteria can be engulfed but cannot be digested or destroyed. Research shows that zinc has a role to play in the prevention of colds, especially if sucked slowly with vitamin C.

- Vitamin C also helps sore eyes and runny nose, as it is a natural anti-histamine.

Most animals are able to make vitamin C in their bodies from glucose. However, humans, other primates, guinea pigs, the Indian fruit-eating bat and the red vented bulbul bird do not. All these rely on vitamin C in their diet and would die of scurvy without it. Man can make very small amounts from folic acid, but unfortunately folic acid is also commonly found to be deficient and only supplied in micro amounts, so we get very little vitamin C this way.

Some scientists believe humans used to make ascorbic acid in sufficient quantities but lost this ability; the mutation did not pose a great threat at first, because we had plenty of vitamin C in our diet. But now storage and processing rob our food of vitamin C, and we eat less fresh fruit than our ancestors did. Other animals, like gorillas, living in the wild, consume about 4500mg of vitamin C daily in fresh food – a hundred times more than the average daily intake for man. Other mammals too, instinctively saturate their blood and tissue with vitamin C and step up their production when they are ill or under stress. It is possible that infectious diseases, cardiovascular disorders, collagen diseases, cancer and premature aging are among the many ills which could be prevented if we still had the ability to regulate our vitamin C levels.

Whilst many studies confirm the benefits of taking vitamin C supplements, others do not, probably due to dosage differences. A useful indication of vitamin C requirements is 'bowel tolerance' – a healthy adult will tolerate up to 4000mg of vitamin C before getting diarrhoea; with flu, this tolerance may go up to 8000mg; while, with cancer or AIDS, it could be 20,000–30,000mg a day. It all depends on the individual, which makes research quite inconclusive.

Age is another major factor: our absorption of vitamin C declines considerably as we get older; though in old animals production is not much different from in their young. Older people need more vitamin C spread out in small amounts over the day.

Which Foods Are Best for Vitamin C?

Foods are listed in order of those that contain the most vitamin C per calorie of food. The figures in brackets are the amount of vitamin C in 100g, which is roughly equivalent to a cup or serving.

Peppers	(100mg)	Papayas	(62mg)
Watercress	(60mg)	Peas	(25mg)
Cabbage	(60mg)	Melon	(25mg)
Broccoli	(110mg)	Oranges	(50mg)
Cauliflower	(60mg)	Grapefruit	(40mg)
Strawberries	(60mg)	Limes	(29mg)
Lemons	(80mg)	Tomatoes	(60mg)
Kiwi fruit	(85mg)	Tangerines	(31mg)
Brussels sprouts	(62mg)	Mangoes	(28mg)

It's worth supplementing more vitamin C during the winter when our need is greater, and supply, in terms of fresh fruit, tends to be poorer. Those who smoke and drink alcohol need much more vitamin C. Smokers, on average, have 25 per cent less vitamin C in their blood than similar non-smokers on the same diet. Heavy drinkers also need extra vitamin C and zinc, as both are necessary for the production of alcohol dehydrogenase, the liver enzyme which detoxifies alcohol.

Aspirin also depletes the body's vitamin C reserves, so these should be replenished by those on aspirin therapy.

Are You Deficient in Vitamin C?

Symptoms of vitamin C deficiency include frequent colds and infections, bleeding or receding gums, nose bleeds, red pimples on the skin, easy bruising, slow wound healing, and lack of energy. If you have some of these symptoms you would be well advised to up your intake of this vital vitamin.

Vitamin C Supplements

Supplements are best taken with bioflavonoids, which help to strengthen the effect of vitamin C. Fresh fruit and vegetables contain both. An ideal daily intake of vitamin C is 500–3000mg; while for those fighting an infection or immune-related disease much larger amounts, up to 20,000mg a day, may be taken. The best way to do this is to buy pure ascorbic acid (vitamin C) powder, dissolve it in some juice and water, and drink it throughout the day, thereby keeping the body permanently saturated in this powerful immune-boosting nutrient. Some people find the more alkaline form of vitamin C, known as ascorbate (e.g. calcium ascorbate, magnesium ascorbate), better. Always remember to take it with a lot of fluid and to decrease the intake gradually when an infection has passed, rather than stop suddenly.

VITAMIN D

When taken in excess, Vitamin D suppresses the immune system. It is, however, essential for healthy bones, and hence for normal movement. The immune system suffers indirectly if your bones are unhealthy and you cannot move freely, because it is muscular contraction that pushes lymph around the body. The immune system must also be suppressed sometimes. After an infection has passed, for example, we need to be able to de-activate the immune system; this requires suppressors. The right amount of vitamin D is needed to achieve this essential balance.

When the sun's ultraviolet light hits the skin, it changes the form of cholesterol in the skin into cholecalciferol, which is the natural form of vitamin D (known as D3) also found in fish oil. Other forms are synthetic versions.

Our skin colour determines the amount of ultraviolet light (UV) we let through and the amount of vitamin D made. Black skin only allows 3–36 per cent of the UV through, and white skin 52–72 per cent. In general, we make less vitamin D in winter because we have less exposure to sunlight. Supplementing fish oil is therefore good for children and the elderly in particular, because bone needs vitamin D for growth and repair (as well as calcium and magnesium). Many degenerative bone problems could be avoided with the right diet, exercise and exposure to sunshine.

Which Foods are Best for Vitamin D?

Foods are listed in order of those that contain the most vitamin D per calorie of food. The figures in brackets are the amount of vitamin D in 100g, which is roughly equivalent to a cup or serving.

Herring	(900iu)	Oysters	(5iu)
Mackerel	(700iu)	Butter	(30iu)
Salmon	(500iu)	Cottage cheese	(2.2iu)
Anchovy	(300iu)	Goat's milk	(2iu)
Whole milk	(41.8iu)	Cheddar cheese	(2.2iu)
Egg	(56iu)		

Vitamin D Supplements

Natural supplements, like fish oil, are best. Vitamin D is fat-soluble and so is stored in the body. It is possible to take too much, so sunlight and fish should be used wherever possible and it should only be supplemented when really necessary.

Vitamin E

Unfortunately, these days we seem to be so obsessed with increasing the shelf-life of foods that some of them last longer than the people who eat them. Vitamin E is an essential nutrient, but it is often removed if the food is to be kept for a long time; although a natural antioxidant, it goes off faster than the artificial ones used to replace it.

Vitamin E is necessary for a normal antibody response. As an antioxidant in our fat layers, it neutralises free radicals and works with other nutrients to improve our resistance to infection. It is very effective in protecting us from air pollution, particularly that due to car exhausts, air purifiers or deodorisers which generate ozone.

Which Foods are Best for Vitamin E?

Foods are listed in order of those that contain the most vitamin E per calorie of food. The figures in brackets are the amount of vitamin E in 100g, which is roughly equivalent to a cup or serving.

Cold-pressed seed oil	(83mg)	Salmon	(1.8mg)
Sunflower seeds	(52.6mg)	Sweet potatoes	(4.0mg)
Peanuts	(11.8mg)	Almonds	(24.5mg)
Sesame seeds	(22.7mg)	Walnuts	(19.6mg)
Beans	(7.7mg)	Pecans	(19.8mg)
Peas	(2.3mg)	Cashews	(10.9mg)
Wheatgerm	(27.5mg)	Brown rice	(2.0mg)
Tuna	(6.3mg)	Lentils	(1.3mg)
Sardines	(2.0mg)		

Vitamin E supplements

There are many reasons to supplement vitamin E. It reduces our risk of cancer and heart disease and slows down the aging process, as well as boosting immunity. These benefits are rarely seen below 100mg (150iu) a day; while, above 400mg (600iu), there also seems little extra benefit to be derived.

CALCIUM AND MAGNESIUM

The mineral calcium is vital for the immune system. It is needed by all phagocytic cells in order to attach themselves to and ingest foreign material. Cytotoxic T cells need calcium in order to make the enzymes which kill. Complement proteins cannot join together to become active without calcium. It is needed to destroy viruses and to produce a mild fever (which enhances the role of macrophages).

Calcium works with magnesium which is no less important for immunity: magnesium is vital for antibody production, the thymus and much more. Deficiency can cause a rise in histamine levels and hence increase allergic reactions.

Although dairy products are full of calcium, they are a very poor source of magnesium. As these two minerals need to be in balance, there are much better dietary sources which are rich in both: seeds, nuts and vegetables, particularly those with a solid structure such as root vegetables. Green vegetables are rich in magnesium but not so good for calcium.

IRON

The right amount of iron boosts overall resistance to infection, but too much is actually bad for the immune system. Iron found in food has low toxicity so iron-rich foods are generally preferable to supplements. Vitamin C enhances our absorption of iron from food.

Iron is essential for the production of antibodies, white blood cells and enzymes made by macrophages and PMNs. It is needed for the detoxification of some drugs and bacterial toxins. Bacteria, however, need iron for reproduction, so it is wise to avoid iron supplements or iron-rich foods when suffering from a bacterial infection. When you have a bacterial infection, white blood cells produce an iron-binding protein to tie it up, so there is no sense in overworking your system at this time.

Iron deficiency is relatively common in pregnant women (probably because they need that little bit more for foetal development) and in children, who generally don't like green vegetables or offal which are very rich food sources. Apart from red meat, which contains the most usable form of iron, wholegrains, beans, lentils, nuts and seeds are all good sources.

SELENIUM

Our daily requirement of this is minute – around 50mcg. It is, however, essential; deficiency is associated with cancer. British soil is very low in selenium so food grown in it is too; and Britain has one of the highest cancer rates. Natural food sources are best, such as nuts and seeds (especially Brazil nuts and sesame seeds), wholegrain cereals and seafoods. Don't however, take regular, high-dose supplements as too much can be toxic.

Selenium helps in the production of antibodies. Research on animals has shown that there is no antibody production at all when the animals are deprived of vitamin E and selenium. It has been suggested that these two, given at the time of vaccination, could increase antibody production and hence the effectiveness of the vaccine. Selenium also helps to produce an important antioxidant enzyme, glutathione peroxidase. And without selenium, white blood cells lose their efficiency in recognising invaders.

ZINC

This is a very versatile mineral, involved in over 200 of the body's known enzymes.

Zinc deficiency causes shrinking of the thymus (the master gland that vets all our T cells), possibly due to the fact that it is required for normal release of vitamin A from the liver, which is needed for normal thymus activity. Zinc is also necessary for the production of enzymes needed for the elimination of routinely produced cancer cells (not for the large amounts produced once cancer is established). The hormone thymulin, which is necessary for T cell maturation, is also zinc-dependent. Like selenium, zinc is an antioxidant. The mineral zinc, in doses of 100mg a day, has also proved to be anti-viral and is available in lozenges for coughs and colds.[2] This level is for short-term use only.

Seminal fluid is high in zinc, so men with high levels of sexual activity need more of this mineral. Deficiency shows up as white spots in the nails and a decline in the senses of taste and smell. Main food sources are meat (especially offal, shellfish, eggs and leafy green vegetables (although Britain, again, has quite low soil levels of zinc and it is not added to fertilisers). Seeds, especially pumpkin, are probably the best source.

MINERALS TO AVOID

Not all minerals are required by our bodies and some are positively bad for us. These 'anti-nutrients' have a detrimental effect on the immune system, either directly or because they interfere with the uptake of useful ones. Calcium, iron, magnesium, selenium and zinc, for example, are often pushed out by the toxic minerals aluminium, arsenic, cadmium, lead, mercury, fluorine and nickel.

The body inadvertently absorbs aluminium (from

packaging and antacid indigestion remedies), nickel and cadmium (from smoking), lead (from car exhaust), arsenic (from insecticide residues) and mercury (from fillings and environmental contamination), even though they can only do harm. Fluoride is often put into British water supplies, whereas other countries have banned this practice. It's also in most toothpastes and used as an insecticide and rat poison. We are getting far too much of it.

These toxic minerals are like keys which fit into the locks of some of our enzyme systems. However, unlike a nutrient, which fits the lock and opens the door, the anti-nutrient merely fills the keyhole so that the proper key cannot be used to open the door. We cannot totally avoid anti-nutrients but we need to keep them to a minimum.

IMPROVING YOUR VITAMIN AND MINERAL STATUS

The first step towards improving your overall vitamin and mineral status is to include vitamin and mineral-rich foods in your diet. Part 5 of this book explains exactly how to do this.

There is also good reason to take an all-round, high-strength multivitamin supplement, plus extra doses of key immune-boosting micronutrients. In a double-blind, controlled trial published in *The Lancet*, elderly people who took a multivitamin halved their number of infections and experienced measurable improvements in the strength of their immune systems.[3] Here are some basic guidelines:

- Take a good, all-round multivitamin and multi-mineral supplement providing at least 10,000ius of vitamin A, 150mg of vitamin E, 25–50mg of B vitamins, 200–400mg of calcium and magnesium, 10mg of zinc and 50mcg of selenium.

- Supplement vitamin C, from 1 to 3g a day depending on your circumstances.

- Supplement an antioxidant complex to bring your supplemental intake of these key nutrients to the following levels: 20,000ius of beta-carotene and vitamin A, 150mg of vitamin E, 15mg of zinc and 100mcg of selenium.

CHAPTER 10

IMMUNE-BOOSTING HERBS

Plants and their extracts, man's most ancient therapeutic aids, are today regaining popularity as effective tonics and remedies. They are still used as the active ingredients in medicinal drugs, such as aspirin, digitalis and morphine. Today, there are several chemicals in plants – alkaloids, phenols, quinones and terpenes – which are attracting considerable attention because of their potential immuno-stimulating or healing properties.

All these herbs and plant extracts are available from health-food shops and some chemists or by mail order (see Useful Addresses). Suggested doses are listed in the chart on page 162.

Cat's claw (*Uncaria tomentosa*)

Cat's claw (its thorn is shaped like the claw of a cat) is a woody vine that can wind its way over 30m (100ft) up through the trees in an attempt to reach light in the Peruvian rainforests. The native Indians have long used its bark to treat cancer, joint problems and many other diseases.

Though still in its early stages, research on cat's claw has been so convincing that the plant has become an endangered species and in 1989 the Peruvian government banned the harvesting and use of the root of the two main species (*U. tomentosa* and *U. guianensis*). It appears that the bark contains most or all of the medicinal properties and grows back after harvesting; whereas cutting or damaging the whole root kills the entire plant. It is still feared that worldwide demand for this bark exceeds the supply so, as with ginseng, the purchaser needs to beware of non-therapeutic substitutes.

Components of cat's claw have been shown to increase the ability of white blood cells to carry out phagocytosis, i.e. to engulf, digest and so destroy an invading germ. It has also been shown to contain other chemicals which reduce inflammation. It is potentially a 'super-plant', with immune-stimulating, antioxidant, anti-inflammatory, anti-tumour and anti-microbial properties.

Austrian researchers have also identified cat's claw extracts which they have been using to treat cancer and viral infections. However, different samples contain different amounts of these therapeutic chemicals, which makes dosage difficult to calculate; it is not yet known whether this is due to location, seasonal or species variation.

Cat's claw comes either as capsules, with 2g being a good daily dose, or as tea (loose or in teabags). Two grams is probably equivalent to two cups a day. You can get more out of the loose tea by boiling it for five minutes and then adding a little blackcurrant and apple juice concentrate to improve the taste.

Echinacea

This root of the plant *Echinacea purpurea* is probably the most widely used immune-boosting herb. It possesses interferon-like properties and is an effective anti-viral agent against flu and herpes.[4] It contains special kinds of polysaccharides, such as inulin, which increase macrophage production. These can destroy cancer cells in the test tube and fight off the undesirable yeast Candida albicans.[5] Echinacea, however, isn't just something to take when you've got an infection. One study on a group of healthy men found that, after five days of taking 30 drops of Echinacea extract three times a day, their white blood cells had doubled their 'phagocytic' power.[6] Whether Echinacea's immune-boosting properties are maintained over a long period of time is not yet known. Some researchers recommend just using these herbs to boost immunity when your health is actually under threat.

Echinacea is best taken either as capsules of the powdered herb (2000mg a day), or as drops of a concentrated extract (usually 20 drops three times a day).

Elderberry

All berries are extremely good for the immune system, as they contain high levels of antioxidants including anthocyans. But elderberries have an extra property, discovered by a virologist, Madeleine Mumcuoglu, working with Dr Jean Linderman (who first identified interferon).

For a virus to take hold, it must first get into body cells, which it does by puncturing their walls with tiny spikes made of haemagglutinin. 'Viral spikes are covered with an enzyme called neuraminidase, which helps break down the cell wall,' says Mumcuoglu. 'The elderberry inhibits the action of that enzyme. My guess is that we'll find elderberry acts against viruses in other ways as well.'

In a double-blind controlled trial in Israel, researchers tested the effects of Sambucol (a specially prepared extract of elderberry) in people diagnosed with any one of a number of strains of the influenza virus. Their results, published in the *Journal of Alternative and Complementary Medicine*, showed a significant improvement in symptoms – fever, cough, muscle pain – in 20 per cent of patients within 24 hours, and in a further 73 per cent of patients within 48 hours. After three days 90 per cent had achieved complete relief of symptoms, compared to those on the placebo who took at least six days to recover.[7]

While this is only the first published trial of elderberry extract, the results to date are very encouraging. Sambucol, which comes as a liquid extract, is available in the UK from healthfood stores or from Higher Nature (see Useful Addresses).

Aloe Vera

Another source of special polysaccharides is aloe vera. While it contains numerous beneficial substances, including vitamins, minerals, amino acids, essential fats and enzymes, its most potent substance is probably acemannan. This extract has been well proven to improve immune power by increasing numbers and function of T cells and macrophages.[8] Aloe vera is usually taken as a concentration of the juice. Check the potency carefully – there's a wide variation – and look for the quantity of mucopolysaccharides (MPSs). Reputable companies will provide this product information.

Magical Mushrooms

Certain kinds of mushrooms have been used for years in China and Japan for their immune-boosting properties. The two most popular are astragulus and shiitake. Astragulus has been well proven to increase T cell count and function and to protect the immune system from radiation and harmful chemicals including chemotherapy.[9] Shiitake mushrooms contain another special polysaccharide called lentinan which also boosts immune function.

Both these mushrooms are available as powders, with the therapeutic dose being 500mg three times a day. However, shiitake mushrooms are now sold fresh in better supermarkets, and dried in most healthfood stores. They are delicious and, as a regular part of your diet, add to your immune strength.

Plant Antioxidants

Plant antioxidants are found in a wide variety of foods which account for the different colours of many plants: for example, purple, red, orange, yellow and green plants all contain different types of anthocyans. Bioflavonoids, found in citrus fruit, rutin in buckwheat, quercitin in cranberry, proanthocyanidins in grapes are all examples of an especially powerful family of antioxidants, anthocyans. Some are now sold separately as antioxidants, including Quercitin and grape extract. Each has a valuable role to play in boosting overall immunity. While there is some value in taking these supplements, we get significant amounts from a varied, wholefood diet. So make sure your diet is naturally colourful.

Herb Power

There are many other herbs and plant extracts that help to boost immunity – Goldenseal, Korean (panax) ginseng, Siberian ginseng, garlic and many more. Goldenseal is primarily used as an anti-bacterial agent. Garlic is an excellent all-round anti-microbial agent, good against viruses, bacteria and parasites. If you're travelling in less hygienic places, it's worth eating a couple of cloves a day to protect your digestive tract. Otherwise, a clove a day is a good addition to your daily diet anyway.

Consider taking the following to build up your immunity:

- A daily tot of concentrated aloe vera juice (as directed on the packaging).

- A clove of garlic every day and shiitake mushrooms frequently.

- Plenty of naturally yellow, orange, red, blue and green foods to obtain high levels of a variety of anthocyans and antioxidants.

- Whenever you're run down or suspect you have an infection, drink cat's claw tea and add echinacea to your daily regime.

- When fighting a cold or flu, take a dessertspoon of elder-berry extract (Sambucol) four times a day.

CHAPTER 11

··

EXERCISE AND YOUR IMMUNE SYSTEM

There are many ways to help keep our immune systems fit and healthy, thus reducing our susceptibility to premature aging and disease. The key to all of them, including exercise, is BALANCE: too little depresses the immune system, while too much is also a powerful immune-suppressor. This is why so many elite athletes get sick easily and are sometimes unable to perform.

WHY IS EXERCISE IMPORTANT?

As explained in Chapter 4, the lymphatic system relies on muscular contractions to keep the lymph moving. Lymph is heavier when it contains a lot of fat, so a high-fat diet and little exercise is a recipe for a stagnant, inefficient immune system. It is known that exercise improves the fat profile of the blood. It also strengthens the heart, decreases the resting pulse rate, and increases our sense of well-being by causing the production of hormone-like chemicals called endorphins.

Vigorous exercise disperses corticosteroids produced during stress; if this doesn't happen, the thymus and lymph nodes shrink, decreasing interferon and T cell production. Exercise improves circulation, thus increasing both oxygen supply to tissues and toxic waste removal.

Trained athletes whose exercise load is carefully matched to their ability have stronger immune systems. According to Dr Michael Colgan from the Colgan Institute of Nutritional Science:

> Trained athletes in good health have a higher number of natural killer cells, and a higher level of killer cell activity than sedentary folk. They also have a higher base level of monocytes. Both animal and human studies show that training programs, carefully designed to provide sufficient stress to challenge the immune system but not enough to overwhelm it, result in stronger immunity.[10]

As the lymph contains a vast proportion of our immune army, it is clearly important to keep it on the move. The human body was designed to move – sitting watching TV needs to be balanced with sufficient exercise to keep us active, not just immune-wise but as a whole. It should also be remembered that too much exercise, as in excessive training, can also suppress the immune system. Everybody is different and requires different levels of exercise. The golden rules are: warm up slowly, stop if it hurts, and try again later. Exercise little and often to start with; build up gradually.

With increased use of technology and division of labour, most of us generally don't do much exercise. We have various joints, muscles and organs that were designed to be used but many of us now follow a sedentary lifestyle, at work and at home. We go from home to the car to the office and back to the car, to the television set and then to bed. This is a very restricted level of movement and not what was intended for us as human beings. Paradoxically, this lifestyle can make us feel very tired and even less inclined to do exercise.

We need a balance in our movements, as in all other things. These days, many people suffer from repetitive strain injury, caused by too much use of certain muscles (usually the fingers and wrists), yet the same people often suffer from other stiff and degenerating joints, simply because they do not use them enough. They sit, cramped up and inactive, using little apart from their keyboard fingers.

WHAT'S THE BEST KIND OF EXERCISE?

Some form of regular exercise (weekly or, preferably, every other day) that increases the heartbeat and breathing to a comfortable, but nevertheless, higher level, is required. Walking briskly for half an hour is fine; if you feel more energetic, cycling, swimming, skipping, jogging, racket sports or aerobic exercise are also suitable.

What Do You Gain from Exercise?

Stamina
Such forms of exercise will not only improve your heart and lungs but also your general stamina – your ability to last without flagging in normal daily life. (Swimming can achieve this, but is not 'load-bearing' so does not help retain bone density which is essential for preventing osteoporosis.) A good form of exercise, if you don't have a lot of time, is skipping: it increases your heart and breathing rate, and is load-bearing. It's cheap, doesn't require a lot of space, and you can stop or start whenever you need to.

Improved Lung Capacity
Lungs age quite rapidly compared to our other organs, usually through loss of capacity, brought about by lack of use. Breathing deeply and properly is vital to stop unnecessary premature degeneration. With loss of lung capacity comes inefficient and insufficient carriage of oxygen to other parts of the body, which can increase the risk of cancer (to obtain their energy, cancer cells switch to anaerobic respiration, i.e. without oxygen). It can also decrease powers of concentration

and increase feelings of depression. For those who are less mobile, singing or playing a wind instrument, or even deep and varied breathing can help.

Flexibility

Next, we need to feel supple – that we can bend but not break. When we don't exercise, our muscles can shorten and stiffen, and lymph flow slows down, causing various aches and pains, particularly in the neck. To be flexible, we need to keep all the joints well-oiled and mobile. Stretching and bending exercises are necessary to achieve this. Massage can also help, especially for those who cannot move easily. (Massage also helps with relaxation and the feelings of well-being associated with touch.)

Strength and Tone

We require strength, not only to lift children and to push and furniture, but to pump blood and lymph around, and to look firm rather than flabby. It is not necessary to do regular weight-training to achieve strength, although weight-lifting is good for this. The aim is not to be a champion strongman, but to look firm, to feel fit and strong, to prevent premature muscle degeneration, and have the strength to do all necessary pulling, pushing and lifting with ease. Sit-ups and press-ups are good for increasing strength, as are cycling and rowing.

In daily life, try to move naturally more often. Play with the children instead of just organising them; garden more often or take up another active hobby. If you don't want a dog, take the children, a friend or even just yourself for a walk. Carry the groceries (unless you only shop once a week and have an unmanageable amount). Take the stairs rather than the lift, and do some of the more strenuous DIY jobs by hand sometimes.

WHAT'S THE RIGHT AMOUNT OF EXERCISE?

Too much exercise can also be bad for you. Intense exercise has side-effects, says Dr Michael Colgan:

> Monocyte concentrations in blood are increased three-fold, indicating a big immune challenge. The lymphatic proliferative response is suppressed, suggesting that the immune system is being overwhelmed by the trauma of the exercise. And the activity of natural killer cells is suppressed for hours afterwards. Because natural killer cells are your first line of defence, their suppression leaves you prey to opportunistic infections.[11]

An illustration of this is provided by a survey which showed that one-third of all participants suffered an upper respiratory tract infection within two weeks of running a marathon.[12]

One way to ensure that your exercise level is just right is to monitor your pulse rate during exercise. The ideal range is calculated as follows: subtract your age from 220. Then work out what 65 per cent and 80 per cent of this figure is. You should try to keep your pulse rate between these two figures while exercising. This way, you do enough exercise to benefit, but not so much as to harm you. As your fitness improves, you will be able to exercise for longer and at a greater level of intensity while keeping your pulse in this range.

BOOSTING IMMUNITY FOR ATHLETES

The more you exercise, the more your body has to make energy from glucose and oxygen, and the more you need to build and repair muscle. To protect oxygen and its by-products, extra antioxidant nutrients are needed. The main ones are vitamins A, C and E, co-enzyme Q10, selenium and zinc. Your muscles also need calcium and magnesium to work so make sure your diet contains plenty of seeds and consider taking supplements of these minerals as well.

The most abundant amino acid in muscle, which is completely essential for rebuilding and repairing it, is glutamine (already discussed in Chapter 8 as a key immune-booster). Taking 5 grams of glutamine after an intense period of exercise, or before bed, helps muscles to repair, recover and grow stronger. However, if you are an elite athlete wishing to shave seconds off a performance record, it is probably better not to take glutamine before an event because it builds up ammonia in the body, which can decrease performance. Instead, you should supplement ornithine alpha-ketoglutarate, from which the body can make glutamine without adding to the ammonia load.

So, in summary, for immune strength you need to:

- Keep active, avoiding a sedentary lifestyle.

- Exercise, ideally, every other day in order to develop stamina, strength and suppleness, and stimulate deep breathing.

- Take care not to overdo exercise; monitor your pulse rate and keep it in the right heart rate zone for your age.

- If you are doing extensive exercise, take extra anti-oxidants, calcium, magnesium and glutamine (or ornithine alpha-ketoglutarate) after a heavy training session.

CHAPTER 12

LIGHT – THE FORGOTTEN FACTOR

Light is one essential nutrient we take for granted. After all, it is the energy from sunlight that makes carbohydrates, our principal food; that keeps us warm; and lets us see. It should be no surprise that light is an essential 'nutrient' for the immune system.

In the skin there are cells known as keratinocytes which produce a very powerful immune-boosting substance called interleukin-1 (IL-1).[13] This rapidly increases the number of T cells by encouraging them to reproduce. IL-1 is stimulated by natural daylight which is a good reason to spend some time every day outdoors exposing yourself, so to speak.

This discovery may explain earlier research by Dr Frick in 1974 who found that exposure to ultraviolet light increases the white blood cell count and improves the body's ability to deal with infections.[14] According to research done in Russia, exposure to ultraviolet light approximately doubles the ability of white blood cells to fight off infections.[15] This finding led to the installation of ultraviolet lamps in factories and schools, to increase exposure during the long, dark winters.

Exposure to natural light is also important because we can make vitamin D – necessary for strong bones – in the skin, in the presence of sunlight. Those with dark skin, living in a country with low light levels, spending little time exposed to natural light (or being covered up when doing so), run the greatest risk of vitamin D deficiency if their diet is also deficient in vitamin D. This vital vitamin is only found in meat, dairy produce and eggs so a vegan is most at risk.

THE DARK SIDE OF LIGHT

Nowadays we are more aware of the dangers, rather than the necessity, of light, i.e. that excessive exposure increases the risk of skin cancer. However, this evidence is far less clear than you may think. In fact, the closer you go to the Equator, where the sunlight is the strongest, the lower the risk of cancer; equatorial countries have almost half the total cancer risk of northern countries such as the UK. This could be for a number of reasons, including different diets and lifestyles. However, it is clear that natural sunlight does generally boost immunity and improve health. (For a fuller discussion of the health effects of light, read Dr Damien Downing's book *Daylight Robbery*, listed under Recommended Reading.)

The only exception to this is those with fair skin, low in melanin, who burn easily and rarely tan when they sunbathe. People with this kind of skin need to be especially careful not to burn in the sun and they do have a higher risk for skin cancer if they do so. Strong sunlight generates oxidants which damage the skin, so you need a good dietary intake of antioxidants from fruits and vegetables to help protect you. These high antioxidant foods are found in exactly those parts of the world where the sun shines long and strong. So nature protects you if you go local. However, if a fair-skinned Briton hits the beach in Southern Spain, lives off fried food, alcohol and cigarettes, and gets sunburnt, their immune system has little chance of fighting off these naturally occurring oxidants.

Interestingly, natural sunlight actually stimulates cell growth but not during initial exposure or the first hour thereafter.[16] This is when oxidants could wreak the most havoc, so we have an hour's grace to mop them up and repair any DNA damage, in readiness for the burst of increased cellular activity following exposure to sunlight.

THE RIGHT LIGHT

Light is measured in two ways: the type of light, known as the wavelength; and the amount of light, its intensity. The wavelength of light determines its colour. Natural sunlight is made up of a full spectrum of different wavelengths which create a 'white' light. Rainbows show the different wavelengths broken up as bands of colour which collectively make what we perceive as 'white' light. Light bulbs are not the same thing. They contain a narrower band of wavelengths and the light is more 'yellow' as a result. Fluorescent lighting is closer. The best indoor lighting, however, is called 'full-spectrum' lighting which aims to mimic the wavelengths of natural light, and its benefits. If you work indoors, with little exposure to natural light, it's worth investing in full-spectrum lighting (see Useful Addresses for suppliers).

So, the moral of this story is that we do need natural light to boost our immune system, but not two weeks of excessive exposure on a summer holiday; rather, a daily or weekly dose of natural sunlight gained by spending time outdoors.

- Spend a minimum of three hours a week outdoors, exposed to natural sunlight. Do not wear sunglasses except when the light is strong. Remove glasses or contact lenses for some of the time if at all possible – it is vital that natural light falls on the eyes. (Glasses change the intensity and spectrum of wavelengths of light.)

- Avoid getting sunburnt by using an appropriate sunblock.

- If you live or work in an area with little natural daylight, consider using full-spectrum lighting.

CHAPTER 13

··

THINK POSITIVE

While your food makes your body, your thoughts make your mind. And there is no question that your state of mind has a profound effect on your immunity. People who (often without realising it) cultivate negative, distressing thoughts are generally more prone to mental and physical illness than those who dwell on happier, more positive thoughts. Researchers at Cornell Medical College in New York have found, for example, that individuals who are frequently sick are those who are more dissatisfied and discontented in general.[17] Polluted thinking can be just as devastating to the body as a polluted environment. Fortunately, however, we do have some control over what we fill our minds with, and can choose the healthier options.

THE MIND–BODY LINK

The link between mental and emotional states and the strength of your immune system is undeniable. Research has now proved that there are changes in immune cell counts, levels of immunoglobulins and immune cell activity depending on your state of mind. The following factors improve or worsen your immune health:

Good for Immunity	**Bad for Immunity**
Calmness	Chronic stress
Caring and empathy	Anger and irritability
Relaxation and meditation	Grief
Laughing	Pessimism
Good relationships	Loneliness
Expressing emotions	Repressing emotions
Job satisfaction	Job dissatisfaction
Tai chi and yoga	Lack of sleep
Music	Noise

One study showed that paying visits to elderly people in retirement homes three times a week measurably improved natural killer cell levels and their overall immunity competence.[18] In another study at Ohio State University College, women who were happily married had significantly better immune function and T cell status than those in difficult marriages.[19] Both intense happy and sad feelings increased the number of natural killer cells within 20 minutes, in a study at California's UCLA.[20] On the other hand, depression, stress, anxiety, hostility and fatigue all result in poorer T cell function.[21] These are a few examples of the growing evidence of the concrete link between mind and body.

Indeed, psychologists now believe that thought and emotion is a 'whole body' experience. After all, immune cells respond to the very same neurotransmitters, the 'chemical communicators', believed to be responsible for thinking.

IMPROVING YOUR EMOTIONAL AND MENTAL STATE

There's much we can do to improve our emotional and mental state. We need to be able to balance whatever life throws at us with constructive thoughts and actions.

Obviously we all have to cope with bereavements, disappointments and pain at times – events that will make us unhappy. Indeed, we need to feel unhappy when sad things happen; we would be very cold and uncaring individuals if we felt nothing at all. But, although we should express our sadness, we should not dwell on these sad feelings all the time. Life goes on and a balance has to be found.

Every day we have a choice: we can make the best of that day; we can scrape through; or we can waste the day completely. The choice is always ours. It is a good idea, every day, to try and do something that you want to do, rather than just things you have to do; to smile; to be enthusiastic; to think beautiful thoughts some of the time even if you are having to cope with a lot of ugly or negative problems. It is vital to believe in yourself, even if you are being put down. Opinion is, after all, only relative. So know and trust your own instincts and abilities and never lose your sense of humour. The fastest and most effective way to change your life for the better is to change your attitude. A hardening of the attitudes can be as destructive as a hardening of the arteries, but it is reversible if you want it to be. If you need help there are a great many personal development courses or counsellors who can help you move to an expanded and healthier level of awareness.

Meditation, Tai Chi and Immunity

Two specific techniques have been proved to boost immunity: meditation and tai chi. Yoga is also helpful, although there has been less research published to date. Stressful tasks performed after tai chi result in much lower production of adrenal stress hormones which, in excess, suppress immunity. Going for walks is also good for your immunity.

So, too, are relaxation and meditation. Meditation has numerous benefits. It has been shown to improve the functioning and number of T cells and natural killer cells, reduce the incidence of illness, reduce the need for anti-depressants among depressed patients, lower blood pressure and, overall, improve a person's health and quality of life.[22]

So, in summary, you can support your immune system in the following ways:

- Avoid prolonged stress. Deal with each situation as an opportunity to learn; keep happy and don't take things too seriously. Laughter is the best medicine.

- Do a job you enjoy.

- Give something back to those around you.

- Make sure you have enough relaxation time – meditate, go for walks, do tai chi or practise yoga on a regular basis.

PART 4

....

IMMUNE
SOLUTIONS

....

CHAPTER 14

FIGHTING INFECTIONS NATURALLY

Lying on his deathbed, Louis Pasteur stated, 'The host is more important than the invader.' It's increasingly being recognised that he was right – we are more likely to succumb to bugs if we are run down; prevention is indeed better than cure. Our best line of defence is to keep our immune system strong, ready for the next invader. We are all exposed to germs that cause infectious diseases, but those with strong immune systems fight back more effectively and either avoid symptoms of the illness entirely or have a milder attack.

If you know you have just spent the morning talking to someone who has the flu, or the person next to you in the elevator sneezed and sent an army of cold bugs in your direction, get in there with high doses of immune-boosting nutrients and start the war yourself, rather than waiting until you wake up with a headache, sore throat and runny nose.

Even if you've missed your opportunity and the bugs have settled in and are stealing your energy, you should still turn up the heat and send in all you've got. Taking it easy for one day in a conducive environment could make all the difference to the severity and duration of the illness, though I admit it would be difficult to ring work with the rather feeble excuse of, 'I won't be in today because I'm going to be ill because of this person I met yesterday. I'll be in tomorrow as long as I get better, but if I come in today I'll definitely be ill tomorrow and won't be in for the rest of the week.'

Back to turning the heat up: immune cells work better in a warmer environment, which is why your body gets 'a temperature' when you are ill. When you have recovered, your temperature returns to normal and the immune cells slow down again (remaining on surveillance duty only). Keep your room warm, and get some sleep. Sleep is the time when your body heals, repairs and produces chemicals which stimulate your immune system. Eliminate other energy robbers such as alcohol, smoke, strong light, loud sounds, over-eating, highly processed foods, stress, sex and over-exertion. Listen to your body – it may not want to eat for a day. But if the illness goes on for longer, some vital nutrients will be needed to replenish the troops.

Drink lots of water to dilute and eliminate toxins produced during the battle and to prevent dehydration. Avoid salt, fatty foods and those which are mucus-forming (dairy produce, eggs and meat). Also avoid concentrated protein foods if you have any sort of stomach upset. A sensitive, damaged stomach could well develop food allergies at this time.

NATURAL REMEDIES FOR BOOSTING THE IMMUNE SYSTEM

Immune-boosting nutrients are good all year round, and especially if you're run down or exposed to people with infections. During an infection both the invader and our own immune army produce free radicals to destroy each other. We can mine-sweep these dangerous chemicals with antioxidant nutrients. These are good for everybody at all times. Antiviral and anti-bacterial and anti-fungal agents are best increased when dealing with a specific invader.

Nutrients	Antioxidants	Immune Boosters	Anti-viral	Anti-bacterial
Vitamin A	*	*	*	
Beta-carotene	*	*	*	
Vitamin C	*	*	*	*
Vitamin E	*	*		
Selenium	*	*		
Zinc	*	*	*	
Iron	*	*		
Manganese	*			
Copper	*			
B vitamins	*	*		
L cysteine	*			
N A cysteine	*			
Glutathione	*			
Lysine			*	
Aloe vera		*	*	*
Astragulus	*	*		
'Power' mushrooms		*	*	
Echinacea		*	*	
St John's Wort		*		*
Garlic	*	*	*	*
Grapefruit seed			*	*
Silver			*	*
Tea tree				*
Artemisia				*
Bee pollen				*
Cat's claw	*	*	*	
Goldenseal				*

THE A–Z OF NATURAL INFECTION FIGHTERS

A – vitamin A is one of the key immune-boosting nutrients.
It helps strengthen the skin, inside and out, and therefore acts

in the first line of defence, keeping the lungs, digestive tract and skin intact. By strengthening the cell membranes, it keeps viruses out. Vitamin A can be toxic in large doses, so levels above 10,000ius are recommended only on a short-term basis, not exceeding one month.

Aloe vera has immune-boosting, anti-viral and antiseptic properties, probably due to its high concentration of mucopolysaccharides. It's a good all-round tonic, as well as a booster during any infection.

Antioxidants are substances that detoxify free radicals. These include vitamins A, C, E, beta-carotene, zinc, selenium and many other non-essential substances from silymarin (milk thistle), pycnogenol, lipoic acid, bioflavonoids and bilberry extract.

Artemesia is a natural anti-fungal, anti-parasitical and anti-bacterial agent, often used alongside caprylic acid for the treatment of candidiasis or thrush.

Astragulus is a Chinese herb renowned for boosting all-round immunity and high in beneficial mucopolysaccharides.

Beta-carotene is the vegetable source of pre-vitamin A and an antioxidant in its own right. It also has the advantage of being non-toxic, although it is prone to oxygen damage and is often unstable in supplements. Red, orange and yellow foods and fresh vegetables are the best sources. Carrot or watermelon juice is a great way to drink this all-round infection fighter.

Bee pollen is a natural antibiotic. It is probably best as a general tonic. Its quality varies considerably, as does its contamination with lead – unfortunately, bees are polluted too. So pick your source carefully and watch out for very cheap supplies. You may get what you pay for. It is best to avoid bee pollen if you're pollen-sensitive or allergic to bee stings.

C – vitamin C is an incredible anti-viral agent. In fact, no virus yet researched in laboratory experiments has survived the onslaught of high-dose vitamin C, from the common cold to HIV. In the test tube, even the HIV virus is eradicated within four days in a vitamin C-rich environment. In a review of research studies using 1–6g of vitamin C daily, Drs Hemila and Herman found consistent evidence of shorter colds with milder symptoms. During a viral infection the trick is to saturate the bloodstream with Vitamin C. Viruses cannot survive in such an environment. Vitamin C is non-toxic. Too much can cause loose bowels though, so, if this happens, decrease the dose to your maximum bowel tolerance level.

Caprylic acid, from coconuts, is a specific anti-fungal agent, primarily used for eliminating the *Candida albicans* organism responsible for thrush. You have to be careful with the dose because, as Candida dies, it produces toxins; so if you kill it off too rapidly you can get worse before you get better. Anti-candida programmes are best followed under supervision of a qualified nutrition consultant (see Useful Addresses).

Cat's claw, officially called *Uncaria tomentosa*, is a powerful anti-viral, antioxidant and immune-boosting agent from the Peruvian rainforest plant. It is available as a tea or in supplements. The tea tastes good with added blackcurrant concentrate.

E – vitamin E is the most important fat-soluble antioxidant. So it protects essential fats in nuts and seeds from going rancid. You'll find it in nuts, seeds, wheatgerm and their cold-pressed oil, but you need to make sure they are fresh. Vitamin E is best supplemented every day with extra during an infection.

Echinacea is a great all-round immune-booster, with anti-viral and anti-bacterial properties. It's the original Red Indian 'snakeroot'. The active ingredients are thought to be specific mucopolysaccharides.

Garlic contains allicin which is anti-viral, anti-fungal and anti-bacterial. Rich in sulphur-containing amino acids, it also acts as an antioxidant. It is undoubtedly an important ally in fighting infections, and garlic-eaters have the lowest incidence of cancer. Consider taking a clove or capsule equivalent daily.

Ginger is particularly good for sore throats and stomach upsets. Put six slices of fresh ginger in a thermos with a stick of cinnamon and boiling water. Five minutes later you have a delicious, soothing tea. You can add a little lemon and honey too.

Glutathione and Cysteine are both powerful antioxidant amino acids. You'll find them in many all-round antioxidant supplements. During a prolonged viral infection your body's stores are depleted and may require extra supplementation. The most usable forms are reduced glutathione or N-acetyl-Cysteine.

Grapefruit seed extract, also called Citricidal, is a powerful antibiotic, anti-fungal and anti-viral agent. The great advantage, however, is that it doesn't adversely affect beneficial gut bacteria. It comes in drops and can be swallowed, gargled with, or used as nose drops or ear drops, depending on the site of infection.

Lysine is an amino acid that helps get rid of the herpes virus. During an infection it's best to limit your intake of arginine-rich foods such as beans, lentils, nuts and chocolate.

Mushrooms, such as shiitake, maiitake, reishi or ganoderma, traditionally believed by Chinese Taoists to confer 'immortality', have all been shown to contain immune-boosting polysaccharides. You'll find them added to some immune-boosting supplements and tonics, or you can buy fresh or dried shiitake in supermarkets or healthfood stores.

Probiotics, as opposed to antibiotics, are beneficial bacteria that promote health and are available in capsule or powder form. They are best used to restore balance in the digestive tract – for example, during a stomach bug. It's best to supplement extra during a bacterial infection. *ABCDophilus*, a combination of three strains beneficial for infants and children, has been shown to halve the recovery time from a bout of diarrhoea. *Lactobacillus salivarius* is a good strain for adults.

Selenium is an immune-enhancing mineral that also acts as an antioxidant. It's rich in foods beginning with 'se' including seafood and seeds, especially sesame. You'll find it included in most antioxidant supplements.

St John's Wort (hypericum) is particularly good for anything that penetrates the skin, such as a wound or skin infection. It's a good general tonic for the immune system.

Tea tree oil is an Australian remedy with antiseptic and antifungal properties. Great for rubbing on the chest or gargling (diluted), putting in the bath, or steam inhaling, it also helps keep mosquitoes away.

Zinc is the most important immune-boosting mineral, well worth upping during any infection. There's no question that it helps fight infections. For sore throats, zinc lozenges are also available.

CHAPTER 15

....

WINNING THE COLD WAR

Are you a favourite host for the cold virus? Do you stock up on boxes of tissues and make Tunes a part of your daily diet when winter comes along? If so, now is the time to strengthen your defences and make yourself virus-proof. There are basically two methods of defence: the first is to prevent infection in the first place, the second is to minimise the effect of infection once it occurs.

Viruses are not technically 'alive' as they cannot reproduce. They can only multiply if they get inside your cells and get them to make more virus particles. In order to keep viruses out, you need to have sufficient vitamin A in your body and enough calcium and magnesium to make your cell membranes strong enough to withstand the viruses.

At the onset of winter, the external temperature gets colder and the body becomes less able to use its supply of vitamin A. This starts a vicious circle, with vitamin A becoming more and more in demand. This is probably one of the reasons why zinc is helpful when you've got a cold because it allows vitamin A, stored in the liver, to be used.

The secret of any battle is to be well prepared. Start now by making sure that you have adequate nutrients to keep your immune system at the ready. Your multivitamin supplement should include at least 7500iu of vitamin A and at least 1000mg of vitamin C as well as a good B complex (one which contains pyridoxine, pantothenate and folic acid). Your multimineral should contain zinc but not copper and at least half as much magnesium as calcium. If you're a person who often suffers from infections you may need to experiment with a maintenance dose of up to 20,000iu of beta-carotene (which is a non-toxic form of vitamin A) and an additional 3g of vitamin C.

IS YOUR EARLY WARNING SYSTEM ON ALERT?

How do you know if a virus has arrived? The first cause for suspicion is if you've been in the company of someone with a cold. Symptoms usually start two or three days after exposure. You also have your own 'early warning system' that tells you you have unwelcome guests: an uncomfortable sensation in the throat or nose on waking; a thick head or a hint of a headache; heavy muscles; feeling slightly tired even before you get up; or feeling hot, cold or shaky. If you feel any of these, don't hesitate to reach for the vitamin C. Even if it turns out to be a false alarm, you can only benefit.

WHY YOU NEED TO TAKE ENOUGH VITAMIN C

Many research trials have shown that large amounts of vitamin C lessen the frequency and symptoms, and shorten the duration, of colds. A recent review of 16 such studies showed that, on average, 34 per cent fewer days of illness are experienced by those who supplement vitamin C. So why do so many doctors still sneeze at vitamin C for colds? There are an equal number of papers that show no effect. A close look at these papers, however, shows two common fundamental flaws.

In some studies, laboratory-bred viruses are squirted up the poor subject's nose. These viruses are so virulent it's little wonder that vitamin C has no effect. It's a bit like testing a boxer's mouthguard by hitting him in the face with a sledgehammer! The more frequent blunder is failure to administer enough vitamin C. The best results have been achieved using between 400mg and 1000mg *per hour*. According to Dr Linus Pauling, 'The amount of protection increases with increase in the amount of ingested vitamin C and becomes nearly complete with 10g to 40g per day taken at the immediate onset of a cold.' In fact, the amount needed depends very much on the person. Some experience loose bowels on high doses, but that is all: there's no harm in taking large amounts of vitamin C for a few days.

In the long term, supplementing 1–3g of vitamin C every day helps keep your immune system strong. It is probably also best to take other nutrients needed to maintain a healthy immune system. One such supplement, Immunade, which provides vitamin, A and E, zinc, selenium, calcium, magnesium and molybdenum as well as 1g of vitamin C, was tested in a double-blind trial at ION in London, involving 37 people. After 12 weeks, 81 per cent of those taking Immunade considered themselves less susceptible to colds, compared to 44 per cent on a placebo tablet. The incidence of cold symptoms and the duration of symptoms were also considerably reduced in the Immunade group.

SEVEN WAYS TO STOP A COLD DEAD IN ITS TRACKS

1. Take 3g of vitamin C immediately and then 2g every four hours (or three times a day) until symptoms subside. Alternatively, mix 6g of vitamin C powder in fruit juice diluted with water and drink throughout the day. Some people prefer to use calcium ascorbate, a less acidic form of vitamin C.

2. Supplement other immune-boosting nutrients, especially vitamins A and E, selenium and zinc.

3. Eat lightly, preferably relying mainly on fruits and vegetables, including foods rich in vitamins A and C, for example carrots, beetroot, green peppers and citrus fruit. Avoid mucus-forming and fatty foods, i.e. meat, eggs and milk products. These make your lymph limp – and lymphatic fluid is the main transport system for immune cells which carry invading viruses to lymph nodes for further punishment.

4. Avoid all alcohol, cigarettes, tea and coffee. Drink plenty of water and herb teas.

5. Boost your immunity with herbs. Drink two cups of cat's claw tea a day, have 15 drops of Echinacea tincture twice a day and, if you have flu or a severe cold, also have a dessertspoon of Sambucol (elderberry extract) four times a day.

6. Take it easy. Do everything slowly and avoid stress. Get some rest and plenty of sleep.

7. If you think you've won the battle, wait at least 24 hours before reducing the vitamins down to 1g of vitamin C three times a day, and one immune-boosting vitamin and mineral supplement in the morning. Once you have been well for three days, go back to your normal supplement programme.

CHAPTER 16

PROBIOTICS VERSUS ANTIBIOTICS

Up to 1.8kg (4lb) of your body weight is bacteria. The average person has around 400 different types of friendly bacteria, mainly resident in the digestive tract, which are forever multiplying. These bacteria are our first line of defence against unfriendly bacteria and other disease-producing microbes, including viruses and fungi. They also make some vitamins and digest fibre, allowing us to derive more nutrients from otherwise indigestible food.

Within every cell are 'energy factories' called mitochondria. The ancestors of these mitochondria, which share the same fundamental design as a bacterium, are almost certainly bacteria that learnt to live alongside the early ancestors of our cells. In time they became part of our cells. So, given the right circumstances; we live in harmony with bacteria.

Like pesticides, the purpose of antibiotic drugs is to kill life (anti-bio). But, in addition to destroying pathogenic bacteria, antibiotics also destroy friendly ones and can damage mitochondria. The more 'broad-spectrum' the antibiotic, the more strains of beneficial bacteria will also be killed. A single course of antibiotics can wipe out beneficial strains of bacteria for six months or more. 'When you take antibiotics, you are doing to your body what a farmer does when he sprays his fields with pesticides,' says medical researcher Geoffrey Cannon, author of the book *Superbug*.[1]

DO ANTIBIOTICS DO MORE HARM THAN GOOD?

According to microbiologist Professor Richard Lacey, the widespread overuse of antibiotics is the major cause of changes observed in the last decade in the balance of bacteria in the gut. Such overuse, in particular of ampicillin and tetracyclines, is resulting in a new generation of 'superbugs' – bacteria which are resistant to the very drugs designed to destroy them. Medical researcher Dr Stuart Levy from Tufts University says that these changes are 'unparalleled in recorded biologic history'. So serious is the problem that there are now new drug-resistant versions of many disease-causing bacteria. Drug-resistant tuberculebacillus, for example, now accounts for one in seven new cases.

Antibiotics also have acute, short-term ill-effects, ranging from rashes to diarrhoea, and chronic long-term ill-effects. The latter are more worrying. Anyone taking broad-spectrum antibiotics continually over a period of years becomes extremely vulnerable to invasion by other organisms such as fungi and viruses. According to Cannon, 'Antibiotics are implicated as a cause of new diseases that are in some way identified with bacteria not normally present in the body. Bacteria that have evolved with us are our outer immune defences, so it follows that anything you do that damages what is a very complex microbial ecology in the body must lay you open to other diseases.' He believes it is unwise to use antibiotics except in cases where there is real reason to believe a bacterial infection is life-threatening or could lead on to more serious illness if left unchecked.

INFECTION EPIDEMIC PREDICTED

It's not just antibiotics, but the whole mentality of developing drugs to kill bugs that needs to be questioned. After all, vast improvements in sanitation in the Western world have been achieved this century, yet in the last 20 years, medicine has doled out billions of antibiotic, anti-viral and anti-fungal medicines. If this approach was working you'd expect fewer overall deaths from infections and fewer cases of food poisoning. In fact, exactly the opposite has occurred.

FOOD BUGS – A GROWING PROBLEM

What of food poisoning? Has this been helped by adding antibiotics to animal feed, or by modern methods of food farming, food processing and storing? More than a million people are dying from food poisoning each year round the world.[2] Indeed, the growing incidence of disease caused by bugs in food, now second only to the common cold in some Western countries may be one knock-on effect of the global use of around 50,000 tonnes of antibiotics each year.

Part of the problem goes back to the post-war years when the demand for meat (a favourite home for pathogens) increased sharply. At this time the demand also increased for cheap animal feed from tropical countries, where animal infection is widespread. Although national legislation and international codes have since addressed this problem, the legacy remains. Animals in Western countries have been given these contaminated feeds, in turn contaminating the environment by enabling micro-organisms to establish themselves widely. Such cycles of infection play an important role in food-borne disease to this day.

The problem is compounded by modern food processing trends. For example, centralised food processing plants mean that a single, infected animal can infect a whole city's meat supply. The decline in home cooking, and the increase of mass catering through restaurants, fast-food bars and pre-prepared meals, have added to the problem. These developments combined with the growing number of people with weakened immune systems and the development of more drug-resistant strains of bacteria, are making the situation critical. High-risk foods are meat, eggs and dairy produce.

KNOW YOUR ENEMY

Contrary to popular belief, most illnesses are not infections and most infections are not best treated by antibiotics. Viral diseases, such as colds or flu, don't respond to antibiotics. Antibiotics don't work for sore throats either, according to a study published in the *British Medical Journal*.[3] Over 700 patients with sore throats were divided into three groups: those given antibiotics for 10 days; those given antibiotics after three days if the symptoms had not cleared; and those given nothing. There was no difference between the groups in the number of people feeling better after three days, nor the overall length of illness.

Many simple gut infections, like gastroenteritis or diarrhoea, can actually get worse if treated with antibiotics. Antibiotics should also never be used to prevent an infection (for example, for the treatment of acne), as they weaken a person's immunity and leave them open to other infections.

Professor Richard Lacey recommends that doctors test whether a sick person has a bacterial infection, identify the type of bacteria, and prescribe an antibiotic specifically designed for that bacterium, for as short a time as possible.

PROBIOTICS

These advances are leading both alternative and mainstream practitioners towards the therapeutic use of probiotics (beneficial bacteria) and away from antibiotics. Instead of giving a drug to wipe out the enemy, specific strains of beneficial bacteria are given to reinforce the body's natural defences. For example, giving children probiotics has been shown to halve the recovery time from a bout of diarrhoea.

The principal friendly bacteria include the families of Lactobacillus and Bifidus bacteria. Supplementing them gives pathogenic bacteria less chance of survival. There are many different strains, some of which actually live in the gut, while others simply 'pass through' and play a useful role while they're there.

The Principal Friendly Bacteria

	Children	Adults
Resident	B. infantis	L. acidophilus
	B. bifidum	B. Bacterium
		L. salivarius
		Enteroccocci
Passing Through	L. Bulgaricus	L. casei (from cheese)
	S. thermophilus	S. thermophilus
		L. salivarius
		L. Bulgaricus

Key

B = Bifidobacteria L = Lactobacillus S = Streptococcus

Those that are resident, sometimes called 'human strain', are usually more powerful at fighting infection. Others are available in fermented foods, such as live yoghurt, miso and sauerkraut. Healthfood stores stock probiotic supplements, many of which contain a combination. Ask for advice on the best one to take, depending on your circumstances. Generally, you need to take 1 or 2 capsules, or a teaspoon a day, providing around a billion individual bacteria. It's best to take them with food if the bacteria are micro-encapsulated; otherwise take them at the same time before or after meals to minimise their destruction from gastric acid in the stomach.

As a general rule, if an infection has persisted for more than a week and has not responded to these combinations, do see your doctor. In some cases antibiotics are necessary but they should only be used as a last resort. If they are, be sure to take a course of probiotics, such as Lactobacillus acidophilus or Bifidus, for one month afterwards to restore your healthy gut bacteria.

If you are going on holiday in a place where you know hygiene standards are likely to be low (e.g. India), take a pro-biotic supplement daily to build up your beneficial bacteria.

CHAPTER 17

VACCINATIONS – ARE THEY REALLY NECESSARY?

One of the million-dollar questions in immunity is whether or not to vaccinate children against diseases, from measles to meningitis. Vaccinations have been hailed as a triumph of modern medicine versus nature. They are based on the idea of introducing a dead or disabled infectious agent into a person and allowing their immune system to respond and produce antibodies. 'Memorising' the antigen, and how to make the antibody gives the immune system a head start in dealing with such an infection should the person become exposed to the agent again, because it can act quickly. The orthodox view is that vaccinations are essential, save lives, have few disadvantages, and are responsible for the decrease in deaths from such infectious diseases.

This view is, however, highly questionable. One of the best reviews of the facts about immunisation is Lynne McTaggart's book, *What Doctors Don't Tell You*,[4] in which she explodes the following myths surrounding vaccinations:

1 Diseases haven't been eliminated purely as a result of vaccination

Many epidemic viral or bacterial diseases come in cycles and have declined due to improvements in sanitation and isolation of those people infected with the disease. A case in point is the Victorian smallpox epidemic in England. An outbreak from 1870 to 1872 claimed 44,000 lives even though most of the population had been vaccinated. The town of Leicester therefore decided against vaccination on the grounds that it didn't work. Vaccines were, however, much cruder then than they are now. During the next outbreak, in 1892, Leicester relied only on sanitation and isolation; there were 19 cases and one death per 100,000. Warrington had six times as many cases and 11 times the death rate, although 99 per cent of its population had been vaccinated.[5]

Despite the introduction of vaccination, the incidence of many infectious diseases continues to rise and fall seemingly regardless. In the US, for example, the incidence of measles continued to rise until 1990, despite the introduction of the vaccine in 1957.

2 The diseases you are vaccinated against aren't necessarily life-threatening

Vaccinations are available for measles, whooping cough, mumps, polio, rubella, hepatitis, tetanus, diphtheria, tuberculosis and meningitis. Some of these diseases are more life-threatening than others. Measles and mumps are rarely life-threatening except in poorly nourished infants with compromised immune systems. Diphtheria – which has all but disappeared – is, however, more life-threatening.

So, when considering vaccination, it's worth knowing how common a disease is in your part of the world and how common death or permanent damage is as a result of infection.

3 Vaccinations won't necessarily protect you anyway

Of course, the popular understanding is that if you've had the vaccination you are immune to the disease. But some vaccines work better than others and some last longer than others. There is also enormous variation between people as to how effective the vaccination is at producing sufficient antibodies. Vaccinations are for particular strains of microbes

Disease Prevalence and Mortality in England and Wales (1996)

Infection	Incidence per 100,000	Deaths per 100,000
measles	11	0
whooping cough	5	0
mumps	3	0
polio	<1	0
rubella	17	0
hepatitis	5	3
tetanus	<1	0
diphtheria	<1	0
tuberculosis	11	1
meningitis	5	5

(Source: Office for National Statistics Monitor MB2 97/3 – Infectious Diseases; < = less than)

which keep evolving and changing, so there's no guarantee of protection. For example, an outbreak of polio occurred in Taiwan, where 98 per cent of young children had been immunised.[6] In 1961, an outbreak in Massachusetts resulted in more cases of polio-induced paralysis among those who had been vaccinated than those who had not.[7]

4 Vaccinations aren't without side-effects

Perhaps most contentious of all, is the questions of side-effects and, in some cases, permanent damage or death as a result of vaccination. Two of the most common vaccinations – MMR (measles, mumps and rubella) and DPT (diphtheria, whooping cough and tetanus) – were thoroughly investigated by the US Centers for Disease Control and Prevention. In monitoring 500,000 children across the US after vaccination, 34 major side-effects were identified; the most common was seizures. The day after a DPT shot, children were three times more likely to have a fit; from MMR, 2.7 times higher after four to seven days and 3.3 times higher after eight to 14 days.

One of the most dangerous is the whooping cough vaccine which accounts for over half the reported reactions to vaccinations. Whooping cough is rarely deadly among well-nourished children so there is a serious question here as to whether its benefits outweigh its known risks. In some cases DPT reactions result in permanent neurological damage (one in 40,000 children vaccinated) and even death. According to research at the Churchill Hospital in Oxford, a child vaccinated against whooping cough is 50 per cent more likely to develop asthma or allergies later in life. This is thought to be because the whooping cough vaccine promotes an abnormally strong immune response to potential allergens such as pollen. Having antiobiotics in the first two years of life also increased the risk. The antibiotics, in turn, damage the gut and may disturb early immune programming.

No one yet knows the combined risks of having a number of vaccinations. It is likely, however, that reactions are more likely in a child who has poor reserves to restore balance after his immune system has been forced to react to the threat of an invading organism. In immune-compromised children vaccinations may overload their immune systems, resulting in toxins affecting the nervous system and brain that the body cannot deal with.

ALTERNATIVES TO VACCINATION

The alternative to vaccination is to ensure that you or your child has a fighting fit immune system. There is no better way to strengthen an infants immunity than by breast-feeding. Once weaned, you need to ensure that the child has an optimal intake of immune-boosting nutrients. Vitamin A, for example, offers protection against measles and probably polio. In under-developed countries, deaths from measles are virtually eliminated by ensuring an adequate intake of vitamin A. It is highly likely, although not yet proven, that a good all-round intake of immune-boosting vitamins, minerals, amino acids and essential fats can turn a potentially life-threatening virus into a mild and temporary illness.

Another way to minimise risk in babies (whose immune systems are immature) is to restrict their early exposure to large numbers of other potentially infected infants in daycare centres until the age of three, when their immune systems are much stronger.

Although less well researched, you may wish to investigate homoeopathic immunisations. In one study 18,000 children were successfully protected against meningitis with a homeopathic remedy, without a single side-effect.[8]

CHAPTER 18

HOW TO BEAT CANDIDA

The name Candida albicans means 'sweet and white', suggesting something delicate and pure, but in reality Candida albicans is a minute microbe, a yeast, which multiplies, migrates and releases toxins. It can afflict us with innumerable symptoms, both physical and mental – bowel problems, allergies, hormone dysfunction, skin complaints, joint and muscle pain, thrush, infections and emotional disorders. Unfortunately, many of these symptoms mimic those of other diseases and are therefore frequently misdiagnosed.

People who suffer at the hands of this microbe often personify Candida as an enemy, against whom they must engage in long and determined battle. The only certain way to victory is to understand its tactics and take the offensive with all guns blazing. This enemy will lose no opportunity to regain lost ground, so the battle must be unrelenting until at last it is won – and even then there is the danger of a false treaty.

This distressing situation is largely man-made. We eat a lot of refined sugar which yeast loves; antibiotics used indiscriminately reduce friendly bacteria and create more room in the intestines for pathogenic microbes; steroid drugs and hormone treatments depress the immune system so that it cannot fight effectively; the formulae in babies' bottles create an early imbalance in bowel ecology. Candida cannot take all the blame; we give it every encouragement. The first stage in fighting back is therefore to start taking personal responsibility for our health.

Obviously, it is important to ensure that the enemy is correctly identified. Dr William Crook published a questionnaire in his book, *The Yeast Connection*, which can help ascertain the presence or severity of an excess growth of Candida. If it shows a high score, and if doctors have failed to make any other diagnosis, it makes sense to embark on an anti-Candida campaign, with the support of a nutrition consultant.

The Candida Questionnaire

History

- Have you ever taken tetracycline or other antibiotics for a month or longer?

- Have you, at any time in your life, taken other 'broad-spectrum' antibiotics for respiratory, urinary or other infections (for two months or longer, or in shorter courses four or more times in a one-year period)?

- Have you, at any time in your life, been bothered by persistent prostatitis, vaginitis or other problems affecting your reproductive organs?

- Have you taken birth control pills for more than two years?

- Have you taken cortisone-type drugs for more than a month?

- Does exposure to perfumes, insecticides, cigarette smoke and other chemicals provoke noticeable symptoms?

- Are your symptoms worse on damp, muggy days or in mouldy places?

- Do you have athlete's foot, ringworm, 'jock itch' or other chronic fungal infections of the skin or nails?

- Do you crave sugar, bread or alcoholic beverages?

Score 2 points for each 'yes' answer.

Symptoms

- Do you often experience fatigue or lethargy?
- Do you ever have the feeling of being 'drained'?
- Do you suffer from depression?
- Do you have a poor memory?
- Do you ever experience feeling 'spacey' or 'unreal'?
- Do you suffer from an inability to make decisions?
- Do you experience numbness, burning or tingling?
- Do you ever get headaches or migraines?
- Do you suffer from muscle aches?
- Do you have muscle weakness or paralysis?
- Do you have pain and/or swelling in your joints?
- Do you suffer from abdominal pain?
- Do you get constipation and/or diarrhoea?
- Do you suffer from bloating, belching or intestinal gas?
- Do you have troublesome vaginal burning, itching or discharge?
- Do you suffer from prostatitis or impotence?
- Do you ever experience a loss of sexual desire or feeling?
- Do you suffer from endometriosis or infertility?
- Do you have cramps or other menstrual irregularities?
- Do you get premenstrual tension?
- Do you ever have attacks of anxiety or crying?
- Do you suffer from cold hands or feet and/or chilliness?
- Do you get shaky or irritable when hungry?

Score 1 point for each 'yes' answer.

Add up your total score.

If you score above 30 there's a strong likelihood that you have candidiasis. If you score above 20 there's a possibility that you have a degree of candidiasis. We recommend that you see a nutrition consultant and have the appropriate tests to find out if candidiasis is your problem.

THE ANTI-CANDIDA FOUR-POINT PLAN

1 Anti-Candida Diet

The aim of this diet is to starve Candida. As sugar encourages fungal growth, all forms of sugar must be strictly avoided, including lactose (milk sugar), malt, and fructose (fruit sugar). Refined carbohydrates add to the glucose load so it is essential to use only wholegrain flour, rice, etc. Other substances to be avoided are yeast (bread, gravy mixes, spreads), fermented products (alcohol and vinegar), mould (cheese and mushrooms), and stimulants (tea, coffee). A positive approach to the diet is essential, and we recommend you read the *Beat Candida Cookbook* by Erica White which shows that mealtimes can still be an enjoyable experience!

Candida often brings on cravings for its favourite foods; at these times steely determination is needed to keep to the diet. However, your motivation will be increased by a clear understanding of what is happening. Even when any Candida-related symptoms have completely disappeared, you should stay on the diet for a further year to consolidate the newly corrected balance in your gut flora. Before long, your 'sweet tooth' will disappear, making it easier to stay on a sugar-free diet.

2 Personal Supplement Programme

You will need to follow a supplement programme to help correct imbalances in your glucose tolerance, hormonal status and histamine level, and to cleanse your body of pollutants. It is important to support your immune system in as many ways as possible in order to fight back against Candida. The situation should be monitored and the programme reassessed at three-monthly intervals.

In an otherwise carefully calculated programme of

nutrients, you can take Vitamin C to bowel tolerance levels to help rid your body of toxins. In addition, pantothenic acid (vitamin B5), 500mg, twice a day, may further reduce the adverse effects of these toxins.

3 Anti-fungal Supplements

One of the most useful anti-fungal agents is caprylic acid, a fatty acid which occurs naturally in coconuts. Its great advantage is that it does not adversely affect beneficial organisms. It is fat-soluble, so it will penetrate cell membranes. As calcium and magnesium caprylate, it survives digestive processes and is able to reach the colon. For reasons yet to be discussed, it is essential to start with a low dose and build up slowly (a process facilitated by different-strength capsules).

Artemisia is a herb with broad-spectrum anti-fungal properties; it acts against a wide variety of pathogens without disturbing friendly microbes. A high score on the Candida questionnaire (pages 133–4), and a history of illness originating in a hot climate, are sufficient reasons to suspect a parasite other than Candida, and to use a broad-spectrum anti-fungal agent.

Propolis is another natural substance which, according to research at the University of Bratislava, is remarkably effective against all fungal infections of the skin and body. It can be taken as drops and built up gradually. Its anaesthetic effect is soothing for oral thrush, and, as a cream, for painful muscles.

Aloe vera is gently anti-fungal, and is a refreshing mouthwash or gargle as well as an aid to digestion. It can be used as an overnight denture soak (preferable to products which are not specifically anti-fungal). Dentures can be an ongoing source of Candida re-infection.

Tea tree oil is another anti-fungal agent, and, as a cream, can be used for fungal skin conditions. Candida is frequently associated with eczema, psoriasis and acne.

Grapefruit seed extract, also called Citricidal, is a powerful antibiotic, anti-fungal and anti-viral agent. Its great advantage, however, is that it doesn't have much effect on beneficial gut bacteria. It comes in drops and is best taken two or three times a day, 15 drops at a time.

With a bit of experimentation, you can soon discover the most suitable natural anti-fungals.

4 Probiotics

Supplements are needed to carry beneficial bacteria into the intestines and to re-establish a healthy colony. The Americans call it 're-florestation'! The role of these bifidobacteria is to increase acidity by producing lactic acid and acetic acid, and to inhibit undesirable micro-organisms that would compete against them for attachment sites. Tissues densely covered with beneficial organisms provide an effective barrier against invading pathogens.

Lactobacillus acidophilus is the major coloniser of the small intestine and Bifidobacterium bifidum inhabits the large intestine and vagina; it also produces B vitamins. Other helpful bacteria are the transient Lactobacillus bulgaricus and Streptococcus thermophilus, which also produce lactic acid as they pass through the bowel. These friendly bacteria are contained in yoghurt which is therefore a helpful food, provided you have no intolerance of dairy foods. In yoghurt, the lactose content of milk has largely been converted into lactic acid by enzyme-producing bifidobacteria, which accounts for its sharp taste.

To ensure that these bacteria pass safely through the gastric juices, it is necessary to take them in freeze-dried form in a capsule. Two capsules should be taken daily, at breakfast and supper, but may be increased to six daily, or even more, in cases of diarrhoea or of illness necessitating antibiotics, which further deplete the bifidobacteria. An acidophilus cream is a beneficial aid for a vaginal fungal infection.

It is essential to follow *all* the points in the four-point plan in order to win the fight against Candida. And there is a fifth vital aspect – support. Anyone entering this 'war zone' will almost certainly find themselves confronted by a host of problems. Confusion and depression are common, and you will need someone who can look at the situation objectively, discern what is happening and point the way forward. This is part of the role of an effective nutritionist.

DEALING WITH DIE-OFF

Thriving Candida releases a minimum of 79 known toxins. Dead Candida releases even more. The resulting general feeling of toxicity can include aching muscles, fuzzy head, depression, anxiety, nausea and diarrhoea. In specific areas where Candida has colonised, there will be an apparent flare-up of old symptoms – sore throat, thrush, painful joints, eczema, etc. This unpleasant situation is known as 'die-off' (or, formally, as Herxheimer's reaction). It has to be recognised as a last-ditch attempt at deception by the enemy – remember that the very presence of the symptoms means that Candida is being wiped out and that victory is imminent.

The aim is to destroy Candida slowly but surely so that it is not being destroyed faster than your body can eliminate the toxins. Initial die-off is usually triggered by the diet (as Candida is starved) and by the increased intake of vitamins and minerals as they boost your immune system. These first two points of the four-point plan usually cause more than enough die-off for most people to cope with. Anti-fungal agents should not be added to the regime until this phase is over. By the end of a month, the majority of people say they feel better than they have for years! Now is the time to add caprylic acid and acidophilus supplements to your programme.

Gaining ground slowly is still the best method of attack.

Most people on caprylic acid can start by tolerating one medium-strength capsule (400mg) daily, without too much difficulty. If, after five days, they are not battling with die-off symptoms, the dose can be increased to 400mg × 2, and so on, up to six capsules daily. After this, they can graduate to 680mg capsules × 3 and increase again if necessary. However, the climb up is seldom straightforward and at some stage there might come a surge in the die-off reaction, necessitating a drop to a lower level, or even a complete break, whilst the body eliminates the toxins. This should not be regarded as a setback, but simply as a necessary part of the process. Drinking plenty of fluid and taking good levels of vitamin C and pantothenic acid, as already discussed, will speed up detoxification. Eventually, caprylic acid does its job and the score on the Candida questionnaire falls to as low as it can, allowing for 'history' factors which obviously do not change.

Slow progress might be due to environmental factors (e.g. domestic gas or mould from house-plant soil) or food sensitivities over-loading the immune system. Avoidance of culprit foods, once identified through allergy testing (see pages 53–4), enables your immune system to work more efficiently. Discovering environmental culprits involves detection and possibly expense if, for instance, the heating system needs to be changed!

Candidiasis is frequently not acknowledged by medical practitioners and may be misunderstood by family and friends. Loneliness and despair add to the physical and mental suffering created by the enemy within. There is no easy way to win the Candida war. It takes courage, determination and perseverance – but it can be done.

CHAPTER 19

....

ACT AGAINST AIDS

Why do some HIV-positive people remain fit and healthy for many years while others go on to develop AIDS comparatively quickly? At present nobody knows for sure, but, after a decade of concentrating on drug therapy alone, doctors are beginning to realise that they may have to look further afield for answers. Research has finally begun to focus on the patients themselves and the state of their natural immunity and resistance to disease. Scientists are considering a range of contributory factors, such as diet and lifestyle, which may be vital in determining whether or not a person infected with the HIV virus develops full-blown AIDS.

It is becoming clear that one very important contributory factor is nutritional status. Malnutrition influences susceptibility to HIV infection and also the progression of the disease. Many studies have found that people who are HIV positive have low blood levels of key nutrients, while those with symptoms have even lower levels. The key nutrients are vitamin C, vitamin A and carotenes, vitamin E, vitamin B2, B6, B12, choline and zinc.[9]

It is likely that these deficiencies predispose a person both to becoming HIV positive on exposure to the virus, and to then developing AIDS. Research also indicates that the actions of the virus result in further depleted nutrient levels.

For example, selenium deficiency is frequently reported in AIDS sufferers.

Whatever the cause of impaired nutritional status, research is increasingly suggesting that improving it may have a beneficial effect on response to treatment and could help people with AIDS maintain their quality of life. The importance of early, aggressive nutritional intervention in HIV infection has been recognised by doctors in the United States, where most of the research has been carried out. A report commissioned by the American Food and Drug Administration strongly recommended nutritional screening of people who are HIV positive and giving them early nutritional therapy, along with counselling and education about diet.

POOR NUTRITION STATUS IS A RISK FACTOR

Recent research, based on data from the San Francisco Men's Health Study, suggested that a number of nutrients might reduce the progression to AIDS in people with HIV.[10] A total of 296 men, all HIV positive, were enrolled in the study which lasted six years. During that period 36 per cent of them progressed to full-blown AIDS. However, the research demonstrated that the risk of developing AIDS decreased, as their consumption of 11 micronutrients (vitamin A, carotene, retinol, vitamin C and E, folic acid, riboflavin, thiamine, niacin, iron and zinc) increased. This relationship was statistically significant for iron, vitamin E and riboflavin and approached significance for vitamin C, thiamine and niacin. A higher intake of all 11 micronutrients was also associated with higher T cell CD4 counts (CD4 is the specific type of T cell most affected by HIV and now considered to be a marker of HIV status); significantly so for six of them. Daily multivitamin use was associated with a reduced risk of AIDS. However, because of difficulties in interpreting the data, the researchers were cautious in their conclusions, saying only that 'the possibility that higher nutrient intakes may delay the development of AIDS cannot be ruled out'.

Another similar study of 281 men from the Washington area found that those with the lowest levels of vitamin C, B1 and B3 (niacin) developed AIDS most rapidly. Also significant was their intake of vitamin A. Too little (below 9000iu a day) or too much (above 20,000iu a day) was associated with increased development of symptoms, as was too much zinc (above 10–15mg a day).

Dr Richard Beach, from the University of Miami School of Medicine, says that patients frequently arrive with very depleted overall nutritional status. He believes it is important to start early nutritional intervention: 'Our studies show people are frequently deficient in zinc, selenium, copper, B6 and B12 even while remaining asymptomatic,' he says. 'In patients with AIDS, nearly every specific nutrient is deficient.'

At the 1992 International Conference on AIDS, Dr Beach reported that 20 to 40 per cent of the asymptomatic patients he studied had abnormally low plasma levels of riboflavin, vitamins A, B6, C, E, zinc and copper. A quarter of them had a vitamin B12 deficiency; they also had low scores when tested for information processing speed and visual/spatial ability. Once their B12 levels were corrected, their performance in these areas normalised.

Other studies have also found evidence of B12 deficiency. Researchers at the University of Rochester School of Medicine found 20 per cent of patients referred for neurological evaluation had abnormal B12 metabolism. They concluded that B12 deficiency may be a frequent and treatable cause of neurological dysfunction in patients with HIV and recommended routine evaluation of B12 levels in patients with neurological symptoms such as tingling or numb fingers.

Dr Beach believes the lack of another B vitamin – pyridoxine (or B6) – can be correlated to decreased immune system activity; he suggests the deficiency is directly linked to the anxiety and depression often experienced in early HIV infection.

THE VALUE OF NUTRITIONAL SUPPLEMENTS

These reports support the value of nutritional intervention at every stage, although conclusive research has yet to be completed. The main focus of current research is on improving antioxidant status. Researchers from the Linus Pauling Institute in California have shown vitamin C's ability to suppress the HIV virus in laboratory cultures of infected cells.[11] They found that, with continuous exposure to ascorbic acid (vitamin C), in concentrations not harmful to cells, the growth of HIV in cultured human lymphocytes could be reduced by 99.5 per cent. A later study confirmed that the continuous presence of ascorbic acid was necessary because when it was removed the virus began to replicate again.

Leading researcher Dr Raxit Jariwalla suggests that healthy humans need a dose of 12g administered orally to obtain the minimum blood levels for anti-viral effect, and much higher levels may be needed in those with AIDS.

Dr Robert Cathcart is an American physician who has been treating immunosuppressed patients for some years. He says that, when a person is ill, their body pool of vitamin C is rapidly depleted and processes that depend on adequate tissue levels (including some for immune response) are at risk of malfunctioning. He is convinced that AIDS can cause this depletion. 'The sicker the patient gets, the more ascorbate is destroyed in the disease process,' he maintains.

Cathcart is a longstanding advocate of large doses of vitamin C, which he says can suppress AIDS symptoms and reduce the incidence of secondary infections. His preliminary clinical evidence is based on experience with over 250 HIV positive patients and it suggests that depletion of CD4 T cells is slowed, stopped or sometimes reversed for several years when doses close to bowel tolerance are maintained. (Dosage is increased until the patient experiences mild diarrhoea and then reduced slightly. This point is known as bowel tolerance.)

The amount of vitamin C which can be tolerated orally by a patient without producing diarrhoea increases in certain disease states such as colds and cancer. However, Cathcart cautions that large amounts of any nutrient should only be taken over prolonged periods of time in consultation with a specialist to avoid induced deficiencies in other required nutrients. The negative effects reported from injected vitamin C megadoses include gastrointestinal disturbances, a rise in serum cholesterol and destruction of vitamin B12.

THE GLUTATHIONE CONNECTION

Glutathione, a tripeptide made up of the three amino acids cysteine, glutamic acid and glycine, acts as a key antioxidant protecting the cells against toxic compounds including heavy metals and excess oxygen. It enhances immune function and is important in lymphocyte activation. It is also critical to the function of natural killer cells and research strongly suggests that glutathione deficiency contributes to the immune dysfunction of HIV, influencing the progression of AIDS.

Glutathione is easily oxidised, unless given as 'reduced glutathione' together with anthocyans which help to recycle it. Alternatively, the precursor to glutathione, cysteine can be given. Again, this can be oxidised, unless given in the form of N-acetyl-cysteine (NAC). Many people with HIV have low levels of glutathione in their bodies – NAC has been shown to raise these. In addition to its glutathione-inducing properties, NAC has been shown to detoxify harmful chemicals and protect the body from heavy metals such as mercury, lead and cadmium, along with herbicides and other environmental pollutants.

It also appears to have other benefits. A study at Boston University School of Medicine, found that NAC could enhance T cell colony formation *in vitro* (in test tubes) and concluded that it might be able to enhance T cell numbers in patients with AIDS or AIDS-related syndromes. Other research has shown NAC's ability to protect against some of the damage caused by radiation, which may be particularly beneficial to patients undergoing radiotherapy for conditions such as Kaposi's sarcoma.

Perhaps even more significantly, NAC was also found to have anti-viral properties. In studies at the Linus Pauling Institute, Dr Jariwalla and his research associate discovered that adding vitamin C to NAC created an eight-fold increase in anti-HIV activity. Recent research has proved that the mechanism by which vitamin C protects against HIV is different to that of other antioxidants such as NAC,[12] this strongly suggests that a combination of high-dose vitamin C and antioxidants that increase cellular glutathione is likely to prove effective.

In the United States, some people have been using NAC since 1988. Anecdotal reports are generally good, though not particularly dramatic. People often report feeling better and having more energy, an effect likely to occur within several days of starting the treatment. The San Francisco-based newsletter *Aids Treatment News* suggests that NAC may be especially useful for certain people with AIDS-related wasting which is not due to obvious problems such as inadequate food intake or gastrointestinal disease.

In the absence of clinical trials there is no recommended dosage as yet. According to researcher and author Dr Richard Passwater, early indicators from laboratory studies suggest that clinically effective amounts may be in the range of 4000mg NAC daily. He cautions that ingestion of 150mg per kilogram of body weight or more may produce adverse effects such as cellular necrosis. 'Appropriate clinical studies need to be conducted to determine efficacy and safety,' he says.

Digestion of fats is frequently another problem area for AIDS patients, and the immune system can be affected by the type of fats consumed. Researchers from the Royal Free Hospital in London and the University of Miami in Florida, as well as doctors in Rome, have all reported depleted levels of essential fatty acids (EFA) in such patients. They conclude that viral disturbance of the metabolism of essential fatty acids occurs with HIV infection and may be a cause of some of the observed symptoms.

In a study carried out at the Muhimbili Medical Centre in Dar Es Salaam, 12 patients with AIDS were given capsules containing EFAs derived from a mixture of evening primrose oil and fish oil. At the end of 12 weeks, the patients had put on weight and experienced considerable improvement in their symptoms, with a reduction in fatigue and diarrhoea and an improvement in skin rashes. Moreover there was a significant improvement in the CD4 lymphocyte count. None of the patients experienced any adverse effects with this treatment.

Approximately 20 months after starting the EFA study, five of the 12 patients remained alive and relatively well, which, according to Dr David Horrobin, one of the researchers, is an unusual survival rate for this region where patients usually delay seeing their doctor for as long as possible.

PART 5

ACTION PLAN FOR IMMUNE POWER

....

CHAPTER 20

THE IMMUNE POWER DIET

On the basis of all the evidence presented in this book, here's how to eat your way to immune health. As well as giving you the basic guidelines for eating for immune power, we've devised some appetising recipes to show you how to put this dietary advice into practice. This is a pro-active diet, giving you foods rich in immune-boosting nutrients, from amino acids to vitamins; while, in Chapter 22, we suggest ways of avoiding immune-suppressing substances.

If you have an infection these are great foods to keep you fighting fit. Depending on your state of infection, though, you may need to give your body a rest from digesting foods. Your body is good at telling you this by removing the sensation of hunger – so listen to it. There's a lot of truth in the old saying 'Starve a fever, feed a cold.' Don't eat while you've got a fever and stick to easily digested foods, such as the immune-boosting soups on pages 151–2, if you're really fighting a strong infection. However, if you've got a prolonged infection or cold, you need to keep your immune strength up.

KEY IMMUNE-BOOSTING DIET TIPS

- **Fruits and vegetables – five servings a day**
- **Seeds – a heaped tablespoon each day**

- **Cold-pressed seed oils – for salads and spreads**

- **Garlic – a clove or two a day**

- **Complete protein – quinoa, tofu, fish, free-range chicken, combined pulses and grains every day**

- **Wholegrains – oats, rye, barley, buckwheat, millet, rice, maize**

- **Shiitake mushrooms – three times a week (unless you have Candidiasis)**

- **As far as possible, eat whole, organic, raw and naturally colourful food**

- **Drink six glasses of water, diluted juices, herb and fruit teas each day**

IMMUNE-BOOSTING RECIPES

Here are some recipes which apply the above principles.

Breakfast Cereals

IMMUNE BERRY BOOSTER

SERVES 1

150g (5 oz) low-fat live yoghurt
100g (4 oz) berries (strawberries, blueberries, raspberries, blackcurrants)
1 tablespoon wheatgerm
1 tablespoon mixed ground seeds (sesame seeds, pumpkin seeds, linseed, sunflower seeds)

Mix all the ingredients together and serve.

OAT MUESLI WITH BERRIES

SERVES 4

4 tablespoons rolled oats
1 tablespoon oat germ and bran
100ml (4 fl oz) warmed soya milk
150g (5 oz) plain yoghurt
2 tablespoons honey
2 tablespoons lemon juice
1 red apple and 1 green apple, washed, cored and grated, but not
    peeled
4 tablespoons chopped hazelnuts
2 tablespoons blueberries or blackcurrants
4 springs of mint
Soak the rolled oats, oat germ and bran in soya milk in a bowl for at
    least two hours.

Stir in the yoghurt, honey and lemon juice, then add the
apples and hazelnuts, followed by the berries just before serving. Garnish each portion with a sprig of mint and a few
whole berries.

SUPER OATS

SERVES 1

25g (1 oz) oat flakes
1 tablespoon wheatgerm
100ml (4 fl oz) soya milk or rice milk or oat milk
1 tablespoon mixed ground seeds (sesame seeds, pumpkin seeds,
    linseed, sunflower seeds)
1 banana, peeled and sliced
1 apple, washed and chopped

Mix the oat flakes, wheatgerm and milk together. Add the
seeds, banana and apple and serve.

Quick Soups and Lunches

WINTER WARMER VEGETABLE SOUP

Here's a wonderfully warming and easy-to-make meal in itself.

SERVES 4

1 tablespoon olive oil
1 medium onion, peeled and chopped
2 cloves garlic, peeled and crushed
700g (1½ lb) chopped fresh seasonal vegetables (e.g. potatoes, swede,
    celeriac, leeks, celery, carrots, broccoli, cabbage)
1 × 400g (14 oz) tin tomatoes
1 teaspoon vegetable stock concentrate e.g. Vecon

Heat the olive oil in a saucepan and briefly sauté the onion and garlic. Add the vegetables, tomatoes, enough water to cover and the vegetable stock. Simmer until the vegetables are cooked.

This soup can be liquidised or left as it is. Use potatoes in moderation if you don't want a particularly thick soup. Add lentils for a thicker, more filling version. For vegetable stew, use less water and don't liquidise.

CARROT SOUP IN THE RAW

Ever had a hot, raw soup? This soup is made cold and then heated gently, which keeps all the vitamin and mineral content intact. It's also full of fibre. Be careful not to overheat it.

SERVES 4

450g (1 lb) organic carrots, washed and cut into chunks
75g (3 oz) ground almonds
300ml (½ pint) soya milk
1 teaspoon vegetable stock concentrate e.g. Vecon
1 teaspoon dried mixed herbs

Place the carrots in a food processor and blend to a purée. Add the other ingredients and process until well combined. Warm very gently in a pan.

RECOVERY SOUP

This soup is also blended raw, then heated to serve. You can experiment with the same principle to invent other instant, high-energy soups.

SERVES 1

2 organic carrots, washed and cut into chunks
3 heads broccoli, washed and broken into florets
1 bunch watercress, washed
75g (3 oz) tofu
100ml (4 fl oz) soya milk
2 teaspoons Vecon or Bouillon vegetable concentrate
tomato paste, spices or herbs to taste

Blend all the ingredients together in a food processor. Serve hot or cold, with oat cakes.

SWEET POTATO AND CARROT SOUP

Sweet potatoes are rich in carotenoids and vitamin E. This simple soup takes only a short time to prepare and tastes delicious. An alternative to sweet potato is butternut squash.

SERVES 2

4 medium sweet potatoes peeled and chopped into small pieces
4 large organic carrots, washed and chopped into small pieces
⅓ × 400ml (14 fl oz) can coconut milk
1 clove garlic, peeled and crushed
black pepper

Boil the sweet potatoes and carrots until soft in just enough water to cover. Purée in a blender, mouli, or food processor, then add the coconut milk, garlic and black pepper to taste.

RAINBOW ROOT SALAD

This colourful combination of carrots, cabbage, parsnip and beetroot is more filling than you may think. Go easy on the beetroot and parsnips, as their strong taste can overpower the carrots.

SERVES 4

3 medium organic carrots, washed and grated
¼ red cabbage, washed and grated
1 small organic parsnip, washed and grated
1 beetroot, peeled and grated
2 tablespoons Essential Balance Oil (see page 71)
1 teaspoon Dijon mustard
2 cloves garlic, peeled and crushed
Lemon juice
Finely chopped parsley

Mix together all the vegetables in a large salad bowl. Mix the oil, mustard, garlic and lemon juice to taste, in a cup or jug. Pour over the vegetables and toss well. Sprinkle the parsley over the top.

Dinners

THAI-STYLE BUCKWHEAT NOODLES WITH SHIITAKE MUSHROOMS

Buckwheat is a wheat-free food with a good protein content. Most buckwheat noodles also contain wheat and these are easier to cook than pure buckwheat noodles, which fall apart if cooked too long. They are best boiled for five minutes, drained, then boiled again.

SERVES 2

1 tablespoon olive oil

2 cloves garlic, peeled and chopped

100g (4 oz) shiitake mushrooms (if you can't get fresh, use dried and soak them)

2 organic carrots, washed and thinly sliced lengthwise into 5cm (3 inch) lengths

100g (4 oz) broccoli, washed and broken into florets

100g (4 oz) marinated tofu pieces

1 teaspoon Thai spices plus 2 tablespoons coconut milk or 1 tablespoon soy sauce

200g (7 oz) buckwheat noodles

Heat the olive oil in a wok or deep frying pan. Sauté the garlic for 3 minutes, then add the mushrooms and toss briefly before adding the rest of the vegetables, tofu, spices and coconut milk and enough water for the ingredients to 'steam-fry'. Cover and turn down the heat until the vegetables are cooked but crunchy. Serve over a nest of cooked buckwheat noodles.

SHIITAKE MUSHROOMS, TOFU AND VEGETABLES

This dish is a great introduction to Oriental cooking. The ingredients can easily be found in an Oriental supermarket.

SERVES 4

1 cube canned fermented red bean curd, mixed to a smooth paste in
  50ml (2 fl oz) water
275g (10 oz) canned lotus roots, cut into 0.5cm (¼ inch) slices, drained
275g (10 oz) canned bamboo shoots, drained
1 teaspoon olive oil or vegetable oil
4 garlic cloves, crushed
225g (8 oz) shiitake mushrooms
1 teaspoon soy sauce
1 teaspoon sesame oil
1 teaspoon vegetable stock concentrate e.g. Vecon
6 pieces of firm tofu, cut into 1cm (½ inch) slices
small bunch of coriander leaves, finely chopped
2 spring onions, finely chopped

Put the bean paste into a saucepan and quickly bring to the boil. Turn the heat down to medium, then stir in the lotus roots and bamboo shoots. Cook slowly for 3 minutes, cover and keep warm.

Heat the oil in another pan over a medium heat. Add the garlic and stir briefly. Add the mushrooms and stir for 2–3 minutes. Add the soy sauce and ½ teaspoon of the sesame oil. Reduce the heat, cover and cook for 2 minutes, then put aside and keep warm.

Pour 50ml (2 fl oz) water into a large pan, add the vegetable stock concentrate and bring to the boil. Add the remaining sesame oil and stir well. Gently add the tofu slices. Spoon the liquid over the tofu and cover the pan. Cook over a very low heat for 2 minutes.

Now take a large plate, spoon the tofu into the centre and surround it with the lotus roots and bamboo shoots. Put the mushrooms and juice on top of the tofu. Garnish with the chopped coriander and spring onions and serve with brown rice or noodles.

SALMON WITH MASHED SWEET POTATO AND BRUSSELS SPROUTS IN A HUMMUS AND MUSHROOM SAUCE

SERVES 2

2 pieces salmon fillet or 2 salmon steaks
2 teaspoons vegetable stock concentrate e.g. Vecon (optional)
2 large sweet potatoes, peeled and cut into chunks
black pepper
225g (8 oz) Brussels sprouts, washed and trimmed
225g (8 oz) shiitake mushrooms
1 tablespoon olive oil
100g (4 oz) hummus

Wash the salmon and pat dry with kitchen paper. Dilute the vegetable stock concentrate in 600ml (1 pint) boiling water in a large saucepan. Leave to cool until just warm. Place the salmon in the stock and bring gently up to a simmer. Poach for a few minutes. Alternatively, grill the salmon under a moderate heat, for a few minutes on each side, until just cooked.

Meanwhile, boil and mash the sweet potatoes, adding black pepper to taste. Boil or steam the Brussels sprouts for 5 minutes. Sauté the mushrooms in the oil for 2 minutes, then add a little water, cover and turn the heat down. Let them cook for 5 minutes until tender and juicy. Purée the mushrooms and add the hummus.

Arrange the salmon, mashed sweet potatoes and Brussels sprouts on a plate, pour the sauce over the fish and serve.

FISH STEW WITH ARTICHOKES AND OYSTER MUSHROOMS

SERVES 4

450g (1 lb) thick-cut, skinless salmon fillet
450g (1 lb) thick-cut mackerel fillet
black pepper
3 tablespoons cornflour
2 tablespoons olive oil
2 onions, peeled and cut into 8 wedges, retaining the root to hold the
  layers together
2 cloves garlic, peeled and chopped
300ml (½ pint) white wine
175ml (6 fl oz) fish stock
225g (8 oz) oyster mushrooms
1 bay leaf
2 tablespoons chopped fresh parsley
12 artichoke hearts in oil
1 lemon
2 tablespoons chopped fresh basil

Cut the fish up into bite-size chunks, removing any bones. Season with black pepper and dust with cornflour. Heat the olive oil in a deep pan. Add the chunks of fish and cook until sealed all over. Remove the fish with a slotted spoon and set aside.

Add the onions to the pan and cook until softened. Add the garlic and cook for 2 minutes. Stir in the wine and stock, the mushrooms, bayleaf and parsley. Bring to the boil and simmer for 5 minutes. (Boiling evaporates the alcohol content of the wine.)

Drain and halve the artichoke hearts. Cut the lemon into thin slices. Add the fish and artichokes to the sauce, then lay the lemon slices on top. Cover and cook for 10–15 minutes. Stir in the chopped basil. Serve immediately with brown rice.

Drinks

WATERMELON PROTECTION

The flesh of watermelon is rich in beta-carotene and vitamin C. The seeds are a great source of essential fats, vitamin E, zinc and selenium. If you blend the seeds with the flesh, the husk (the black part) of the seed sinks to the bottom and the seeds blend with the flesh to make an incredibly immune-boosting fruit drink. This is ideal during an infection as it provides enough glucose for energy, some protein from the seeds and plenty of immune-boosting nutrients. It also provides excellent protection against pollution if visiting a heavily polluted city.

HI-5 VEGETABLE JUICE

There are a hundred and one fruit and vegetable juices that are great for your immunity and health. If you have a juicer, probably the top five which blend to make a great taste are:

175g (6 oz) carrot
175g (6 oz) apple
60g (2 oz) beetroot
60g (2 oz) watercress
60g (2 oz) cucumber

If you don't have a juicer you can buy mixed vegetable juices or combine, in the same proportions, carrot, apple and beetroot juices.

BERRY JUICE COCKTAILS

There's an ever-increasing variety of fruit and berry juices available. Particularly good are loganberries, blueberries and blackcurrants. See what's available in your local healthfood store. Pick pure juices with no added sugar. These are nectar for the immune system, with plenty of vitamin C and anthocyans. They are often best diluted half and half with water to dilute the natural fruit sugars. Alternative, make your own:

300ml (½ pint) apple juice
350g (12 oz) mixed berries (e.g. blueberries, blackberries, strawberries)

Put into a blender and whiz up.

CHAPTER 21

IMMUNE-BOOSTING SUPPLEMENTS

In addition to eating an immune-boosting diet, there's definite value in taking supplements of certain vitamins, minerals and herbs. Your ideal intake needs to match your own unique needs – depending on genetic factors, your diet, lifestyle and environment. The 'basic' recommendations given in the table below are therefore only a guide. For a personal assessment of what you need to achieve optimal immune health, we recommend that you see a nutrition consultant.

In practical terms, the easiest way to achieve these levels is to supplement:

- **A good all-round multivitamin and mineral**

- **Vitamin C (with bioflavonoids)**

- **An antioxidant complex (for A, C, E, zinc, selenium, NAC or glutathione)**

- **Plus 'extras' if you need a boost (such as cat's claw, Echinacea, glutamine)**

Your needs are different when you have an infection, when you are at a high risk of getting one (perhaps because a member of your family is unwell), or when you are recovering from one. Under these circumstances your immune system is likely to need an 'extra boost'.

The 'extra boost' dosages given in the table below do not cover specific anti-infection remedies that you may wish to employ for a specific kind of infection (such as caprylic acid for thrush, high-dose vitamin C for a cold, grapefruit seed extract or probiotics for a stomach bug). For guidance on such natural remedies, and the right amount to take during an infection, please see Chapters 14, 15, 18, 19 and the Index.

It's worth bumping up the amount of antioxidant supplements and vitamin C you take for an immune boost and keeping vitamin C, Echinacea and cat's claw on hand in case of the first signs of an immune attack or simply because you're run down or exposed to other people with an active infection.

While anthocyans (including bioflavonoids), garlic and essential fats all have immune-boosting properties and have real value as supplements, you can obtain more of these nutrients from the food in an optimal diet than you can realistically absorb from supplements.

Ideal Supplementary Nutrient Intake for Immune Power

Nutrient	Basic Prevention	Extra Boost
Vitamins		
Vitamin A	**20,000iu**	**35,000iu**
(as retinol	7500iu	7500iu)
(as beta-carotene	12,500iu	22,500iu)
Vitamin C	**1000mg**	**3000–5000mg**
Vitamin D	400ius	
Vitamin E	**150mg (200iu)**	**400mg (600iu)**
B1 (Thiamine)	25mg	
B2 (Riboflavin)	25mg	
B3 (Niacin)	25mg	100mg
B5 (Pantothenic acid)	**25mg**	**50–100mg**
B6 (Pyridoxine)	**25mg**	**50–100mg**

Ideal Supplementary Nutrient Intake for Immune Power (*continued*)

Nutrient	Basic Prevention	Extra Boost
B12	**10mcg**	**20mcg**
Folic acid	**100mcg**	**400mcg**
Biotin	50mcg	

<u>Minerals</u>		
Calcium	**350mg**	**800mg**
Magnesium	**200mg**	**500mg**
Zinc	**15mg**	**25mg**
Iron	10mg	
Manganese	5mg	10mg
Chromium	50mcg	100mcg
Selenium	**50mcg**	**200mcg**

<u>Amino Acids</u>		
Reduced glutathione*	50mg	100mg
<u>or</u> N-Acetyl Cysteine	500mg	1000mg
Glutamine	1000mg	5000mg

<u>Herbs</u>		
Cat's claw		**1000–2000mg (1–2 cups)**
Echinacea		**1000–2000mg (30–60 drops)**
Aloe vera		as instructed
Anthocyans/bioflavonoids		200–500mg

Most important nutrients are in **bold**

* Glutathione must be enteric–coated to prevent degradation in the stomach. It must also be combined with anthocyans which recycle glutathione, making it much more powerful. Both Rejuvan Forte and Glutathon Forte fulfil these requirements.

CHAPTER 22

STOP THE IMMUNE SUPPRESSORS

Just as significant as nutrients are 'anti-nutrients', substances that interfere with nutrients and suppress the immune system.

Immune suppressors include cigarettes, coffee, alcohol, stress, a negative attitude, lack of sleep and lack of natural sunlight. Put this lot together and you're really increasing your chances of picking up infections.

There are four main ways to tackle the immune suppressors:

1 Go low on stimulants – cigarettes, coffee and tea

Chemicals in cigarettes, coffee and tea work by stimulating the adrenal glands to raise blood sugar levels and liberate energy for the body in times of emergency. In the short term this has little effect on immunity. However, prolonged, excessive use of stimulants leads to prolonged stress which is a powerful immune suppressor. Cigarettes tax the immune system because of the oxidants in the smoke and are therefore potent immune suppressors. Coffee is mild and tea milder still. There is no strong evidence that the odd cup of coffee or tea is harmful for immunity, but frequent, addictive consumption may be.[1]

2 Cut down on alcohol

Of all the immune suppressors, alcohol is the most powerful. Alcohol has been reported to have adverse effects on all major components of the immune system.[2] Generally, two things happen: the number and strength of lymphocytes goes down and the number of circulating immunoglobulins (IgA and IgM) goes up, indicating that the body is reacting to the alcohol. This suggests that alcohol both taxes the immune system and suppresses it. The more you drink and the more often you drink, the greater the effect. So it's critical to cut out, or at least cut down on, alcohol consumption when your immune strength is already low, perhaps from too much stress or not enough sleep.

Cannabis is also a potent immune suppressor, but only in very large amounts. Studies showing evidence of immune suppression generally used levels far beyond those that a person would normally use.[3] However, once again, the oxidants from smoke tax the immune system, thereby weakening your defences.

3 Get enough sleep

Getting enough sleep is vital for the immune system. Numerous scientific studies have demonstrated a profound decline in immunity after either a night without sleep or a continuous period of just not getting enough. These studies show a fall in natural killer cells and lymphocytes. Just one night without sleep can reduce natural killer cell activity by as much as 30 per cent.[4] There is a harmonious relationship between the sleep cycle and immunity so make sure you are getting enough. That means not less than six hours in 24 hours. Less than this, or more than eight hours, equates to a lower health rating in the long term. When your body is fighting an infection you may need more sleep. It's important to rest when you need to, as this hastens recovery and gets you back into action.

As discussed in Chapters 11, 12 and 13, you need to keep moving and participate in regular exercise to stimulate your immune system, while taking care not to overdo it, as too much exercise suppresses immunity. Some daily exposure to natural sunlight is also vital in order to maintain a healthy immune system.

4 Protect your immune system from late-night parties

Imagine you go to a party, stressed after a hard week's work, eat food that you're allergic to, drink much too much alcohol, smoke or inhale other people's cigarettes, and stay up until 3am with no exposure to natural light. All these factors add up to big trouble for the immune system. With your immune defences down, it doesn't take much for a virus from one of your dancing partners to find a new home and settle in.

Our advice is to stoke up on immune boosters, such as zinc, vitamin C, Echinacea and cat's claw, and cut back on immune suppressor overload. This way you can enjoy yourself both at the party and the next day.

All this means that, for maximum immunity, you should:

■ Quit smoking.

■ Cut back on daily, habitual tea and coffee drinking.

■ Have no more than one unit of alcohol a day, and preferably not every day.

■ Stay away from sugar and refined carbohydrates which rob your body of nutrients.

■ Get enough sleep – between 6.5 and 8 hours a night is ideal.

■ Exercise regularly, preferably in natural daylight.

RECOMMENDED READING

Part 2
Dr Braly's Food Allergy and Nutrition Revolution, Dr James Braly, Keats Publishing, 1992

Part 3
The Optimum Nutrition Bible, Patrick Holford, Piatkus, 1997
The Ultimate Nutrient Glutamine, Judy Shabert and Nancy Ehrlich, Avery Publishing Group, 1993
Daylight Robbery, Dr Damien Downing, Arrow Books, 1988

Part 4
What Doctors Don't Tell You, Lynne McTaggart, Thorsons, 1996
Beat Candida Cookbook, Erica White, White Publications, 1993 (Available from the Institute for Optimum Nutrition)
The Yeast Connection, Dr William Crook, Professional Books USA, 1995

USEFUL ADDRESSES

Institute for Optimum Nutrition (ION)
ION offers personal consultations with qualified nutrition consultants and courses including the one-day Optimum Nutrition Workshop, the Homestudy Course and the three-year Nutrition Consultants Diploma Course. They also have a Directory of Nutrition Consultants (£2) to help you find a nutrition consultant in your area. For details on courses, consultations and publications, send a stamped addressed envelope to: ION, Blades Court, Deodar Road, London SW15 2NU, or visit website **www.optimumnutrition.co.uk** Tel: 0181 877 9993 or Fax: 0181 877 9980 (see also p.173).

FSL
FSL supplies a wide range of full-spectrum lighting, including bulbs and tubes.
Unit 1, Riverside Business Centre, Victoria Street, High Wycombe, Bucks HP11 2LT.
Tel: 01494 448727.

Higher Nature
Higher Nature produces and supplies a range of vitamin, mineral and herbal supplements, including Sambucol (elderberry extract), Citricidal (grapefruit seed extract) and Immune Prevention.
Burwash Common, East Sussex TN19 7LX.
Tel: 01435 882880.

Solgar

Solgar produce a wide range of nutritional and herbal supplements available from any good healthfood store including Microbial Modulators. For your nearest stockist, contact Solgar Vitamins Ltd, Aldbury, Tring, Hertfordshire HP23 5PT.
Tel: 01442 890355.

Health Plus

Health Plus produce an extensive range of supplements including Immunade, available by mail order. Send for a free catalogue to Health Plus Ltd, Dolphin House, 30 Lushington Road, Eastbourne, East Sussex BN21 4LL.
Tel: 01323 737374.

Rejuvan forte

This is a combination of anthocyans and reduced glutathione, available in pharmacists. In case of difficulty contact Beauty Products International Ltd, Unit 26, Lyon Road, Hersham, Walton-on-Thames, Surrey KT12 3PM.
Tel: 01932 889222.

Nutrition Consultations

For personal referral by Patrick Holford to a clinical nutritionist in your area, specialising in your area of health concern, please write to Holford & Associates, 34 Wadham Road, London SW15 2LR, stating your name, address, telephone number and brief details of your health issue (for overseas requests include your fax or e-mail), or visit **www.patrickholford.com**.

References

Part 1

1. Report of Cancer Incidence and Prevalence Projections, East Anglia Cancer Intelligence Unit, Department of Community Medicine, University of Cambridge, June 1997, Macmillan Cancer Relief.
2. Berkman, L. and Syme, S., 'Social networks, host resistance and mortality: A nine-year follow-up study of Alameda County residents', *Am. J. Epidemiology*, vol 109, pp 186–204 (1979).
3. Reynolds, P. and Kaplan, G., 'Social connections and cancer: A prospective study of Alameda County residents', Paper presented at the annual meeting of the Society of Behavioural Medicine, San Francisco (March 1986).
4. Department of Health, Prescription Cost Analysis (1996).
5. *New Scientist* (17 Dec. 1994).

Part 3

1. Harakeh, S. et al., 'Suppression of human immunodeficiency virus replication by ascorbate in chronically and acute infected cells', *Proc. Natl. Acad. Sci.*, vol 87, pp 7245–49 (Sept. 1990).
2. Godfrey, J. et al., 'Zinc for treating the common cold: review of all clinical trials since 1984', *Altern. Ther.*, vol 2(6), pp 63–72 (1996).
3. Chandra R., 'Effect of vitamin and trace element supplementation on immune responses and infection in elderly subjects', *Lancet*, vol 340, pp 1124–27 (1992).

4. *Br. J. Phytotherapy*, vol 2, p 2 (1991).

5. Roesler, J et al., 'Application of purified polysaccharides from cell cultures of the plant Echinacea purpurea to mice mediates protection against systemic infections with Listeria monocytogenes and Candida albicans', *Int. J. Immunopharmac.*, vol 13, pp 27–37 (1991).

6. Erhard, M. et al., 'Effect of Echinacea, Aconitum, Lachesis and Apis extracts, and their combinations on phagocytosis of human granulocytes', *Phytother. Res.*, vol 8, pp 14–17 (1994).

7. Zakay-Rones, Z. et al., 'Inhibition of several strains of influenza virus in vitro and reduction of symptoms by an elderberry extract (Sambucus nigra L.) during an outbreak of influenza B Panama', *J. Alt. and Comp. Med.*, vol 1, pp 361–9 (1995).

8. Womble, D. and Helderman, J., 'Enhancement of allo-responsiveness of human lymphocytes by acemannan (Carrisyn)', *Int. J. Immunopharmac.*, vol 10, pp 967–74 (1988).

Hart, L. et al., 'Effects of low molecular constituents from Aloe vera gel on oxidative metabolism and cytotoxic and bactericidal activities of human neutrophils', *Int. J. Immunopharmac.*, vol 12, pp 427–34 (1990).

9. Zhao, K. et al., 'Enhancement of the immune response in mice by Astragulus membranaceus,' *Immunopharmacol.*, vol 20, pp 225–33 (1990).

Chu, D. et al., 'Immunotherapy with Chinese and medicinal herbs, I: Immune restoration of local xenogenic graft–versus–host reaction in cancer patients by fractionated Astragulus membranaceus in vitro', *J. Clin. Lab. Immunol.*, vol 25, pp 119–23 (1988).

10. Colgan, Dr Michael, *Optimum Sports Nutrition*, Advanced Research Press, New York (1993).

11. Colgan, as above.

12. Peters, E. and Bateman, E., 'Ultra-marathon running and upper respiratory tract infection – an epidemiological survey', *South African Med. J.*, vol 64, pp 582–4 (1983).

13. Downing, D., *Daylight Robbery*, Arrow Books Limited, pp 58–9 (1988).

14. Frick, Dr G., 'Zur wirkung der Ultravioletbestrahlung des Blutes auf das Blutbild', *Folia Haematol.*, vol 101, pp 871–7 (1974).

15. Zabaluyera, A., 'General immunological reactivity of the organism to prophylactic UN irradiation of children in Northern regions', *Vestn. Akad. Med. Nank. SSSR*, vol 3, pp 23 (1975).

16. Pathak, M., 'Activation of the Melanocyte System by Ultraviolet Radiation and Cell Transformation', *Ann. NY Acad. Sci.* vol 453, pp 328–39 (1985).

17. Hinkle, L. and Wolff, H., 'Ecologic investigation of the relationship between illness, life experiences and the social environment', *Ann. Int. Med.*, vol 49, pp 1373–88 (1958).

18. Kiecolt-Glaser, J. et al., 'The enhancement of immune competence by relaxation and social contact', Paper presented at the annual meeting of the Society of Behavioural Medicine, Philadelphia (May 1984).

19. Kiecolt-Glaser, J., 'Clinical psychoneuroimmunology in health and disease: Effects of marital quality and disruption', Paper presented at the annual meeting of the Society of Behavioural Medicine, San Francisco (March 1986).

20. Kemeny, M., 'Emotions and the immune system', in Moyers, B., *Healing and the Mind*, pp 195–211, Doubleday, New York (1993).

21. Kemeny, M., 'Psychological and immunological prediction of recurrence in Herpes simplex II', *Psychosomatic Med.*, vol 51, pp 195–208 (1989).

22. Magarey, C., 'Meditation and Health', *Darshan magazine* SYDA Foundation, NY 12779, USA (Sept. 1993).

Part 4

1. Cannon, G., *Superbug*, Virgin Publishing (1995).

2. *New Scientist* (17 Dec. 1994).

3. Little, P. et al., 'Open randomised trial of prescribing strategies in managing sore throat,' *BMJ*, vol 8; 314(7082), pp 722–7 (Mar. 1997).

4. McTaggart, L., *What Doctors Don't Tell You*, Ch. 6, Thorsons (1996).

5. 'Campaign Against Fraudulent Medical Research Newsletter', vol 2(3), pp 5–13 (1995), quoting statistics from the London Bills of Mortality 1760–1834 and Reports of the Registrar General 1838–96, as compiled in Alfred Wallace, *The Wonderful Century* (1898).

6. *The Lancet*, vol 344, pp 630–1 (1994).

7. Walene, James, *Immunization: The Reality Behind the Myth*, Bergin & Garvey, Massachusetts (1988).

8. *BMJ*, vol 294, pp 294–6 (1987).

9. Jariwalla, R., 'Micronutrient imbalance in HIV infection and AIDS,' *J. Nut. Med.*, vol 5, pp 297–306 (1995).

10. Abrams, B. et al., 'A prospective study of dietary intake and acquired immune deficiency syndrome in HIV-seropositive homosexual men,' *J. AIDS*, vol 6, pp 949–58 (1993).

11. Harekeh, S. and Jariwalla, R., 'Suppression of human immunodeficiency virus replication by ascorbate in chronically and acutely infected cells,' *Proc. Natl. Acad. Sci.*, vol 87, pp 7245–9, USA (1990).

12. Harakeh, S. and Jariwalla, R., 'NFkB-Independent suppression of HIV expression by ascorbic acid, *AIDS Res.*, vol 13(3), pp 235–9 (1997).

Part 5

1. Melamed, I. et al., 'Coffee and the immune system,' *Int. J. Immunopharmacol.*, vol 12(1), pp 129–34 (1990).

2. Baker, R. and Jerrells, T., 'Recent developments in alcoholism: immunological aspects,' *Recent Dev. Alcohol*, vol 11, pp 249–71 (1993).

Mili, F. et al., 'The associations of alcohol drinking and drinking cessation with measures of the immune system in middle-aged men,' *Alcohol Clin. Exp. Res.*, vol 16(4), pp 688–94 (1992).

3. Hollister, L., 'Marijuana and immunity', *J. Psychoactive drugs*, vol 24(2), pp 159–64 (1992).

4. Irwin, M. et al., 'Partial night sleep deprivation reduces natural killer and cellular immune responses in human,' *FASEB J.*, vol 10(5), pp 643–53 (Apr. 1996).

Moldofsky, H. et al., 'Effects of sleep deprivation on human immune functions,' *FASEB J.*, vol 3(8), pp 1972–7 (Jun. 1989).

Born, J. et al., 'Effects of sleep and circadian rhythm on human circulating immune cells,' *J. Immunol.*, vol 158(9), pp 4454–64 (1 May 1997).

Moldofsky, H., 'Central nervous system and peripheral immune functions and the sleep-wake system,' *J. Psychiatry Neurosci.*, vol 19(5), pp 368–74 (Nov. 1994).

INDEX